THE Plant-Based DIABETES COOKBOOK

THE Plant-Based DIABETES COOKBOOK

125+ Nourishing Recipes to Satisfy Every Taste Bud

JACKIE NEWGENT, RDN, CDN

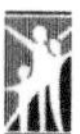

Health Communications, Inc.
Boca Raton, Florida
www.hcibooks.com

Library of Congress Cataloging-in-Publication Data
is available through the Library of Congress

ISBN-13: 978-07573-2482-6 (Paperback)
ISBN-10: 07573-2482-7 (Paperback)
ISBN-13: 978-07573- 2483-3 (ePub)
ISBN-10: 07573-2483-5 (ePub)

Publisher: Health Communications, Inc.
301 Crawford Blvd., Suite 200
Boca Raton, FL 33432-3762

Cover and interior design and formatting by Larissa Hise Henoch

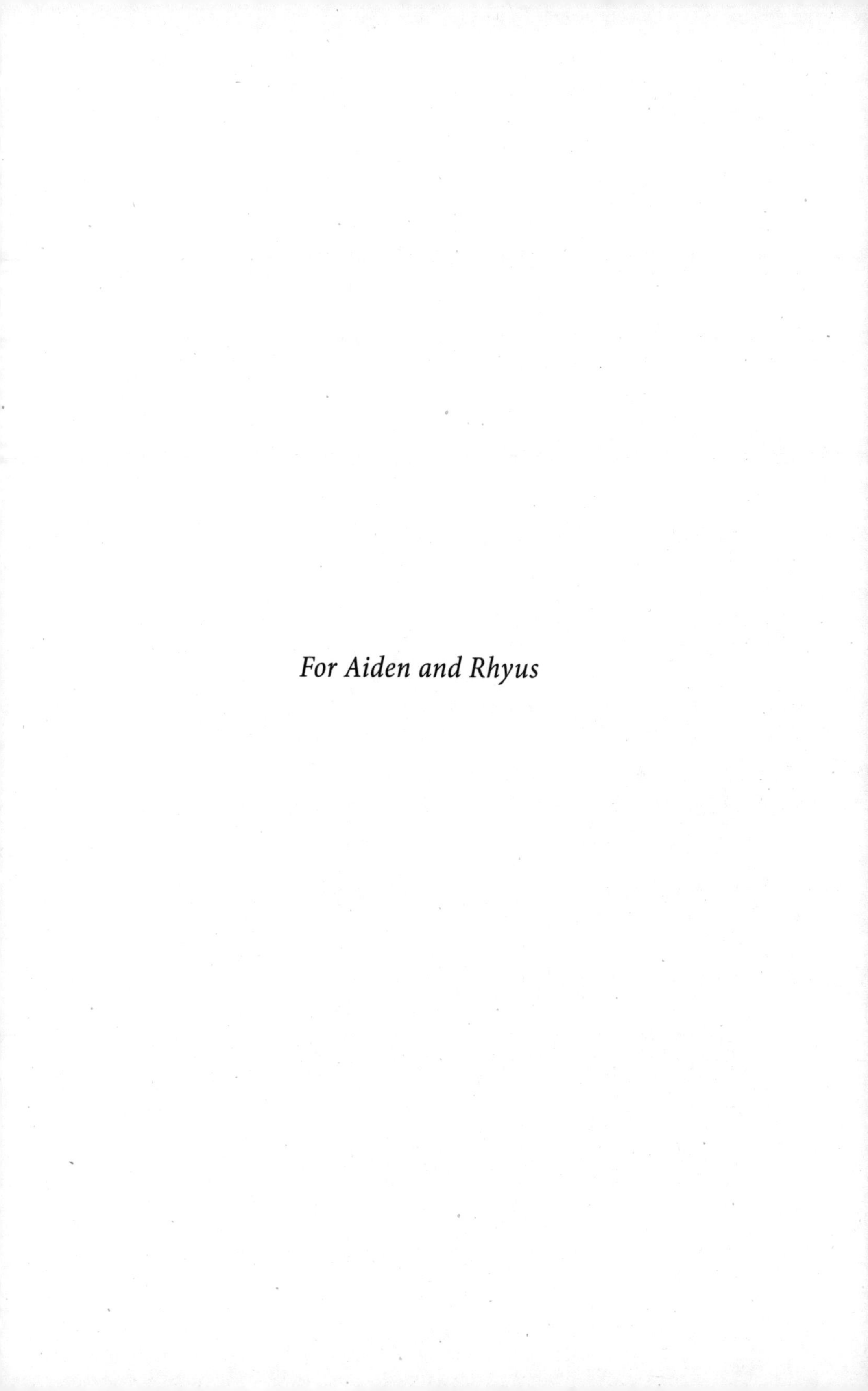

For Aiden and Rhyus

Contents

Acknowledgments

Many inspiring and brainy people have helped make this cookbook possible. I'm grateful to have the opportunity to thank them here for their generosity, time, commitment, passion, energy, and support.

THANK YOU!

- Jim, Sandi, Aiden, and Rhyus Newgent, and Rebecca, Don, and Jaime McLean, for being my favorite tasters and biggest fans.
- My dear friends—you all know who you are—for your never-ending love and understanding . . . and for nibbling up my leftovers.
- Linda Konner, for your cheerful and determined guidance as my agent.
- Megan Warnke, RDN, CDCES, for your expertise in diabetes nutrition.
- All of the dedicated and creative talent at Health Communications, Inc., including Christine Belleris, Christian Blonshine, Larissa Henoch, and Lindsey Mach.
- Baby Duke (my cat!), for being a constant source of entertainment and my eager "sous chef."

Introduction

Today, we know that deliciousness can and should be part of any eating plan for diabetes. And the current nutritional guidance for diabetes is smarter than ever.

What's in? Individualization. What's out? Strictness. Nutrition therapy guidelines are now flexible and personal, versus being overly focused on calories, carb counting, or other precise macronutrient or micronutrient parameters. While there are some people who will still need to follow a more detailed plan, that's no longer the standard for many people with type 2 diabetes. Hooray for that!

Ultimately, diabetes is a condition that you can live with and manage happily, scrumptiously, and simply. One of the most nourishing ways to do that is by following a plant-based eating approach.

That's where *The Plant-Based Diabetes Cookbook: 125+ Nourishing Recipes to Satisfy Every Taste Bud* comes in. The recipes in this book will appeal to anyone who wishes to eat more plants and do so wholesomely. While the dishes are all 100 percent plant-based (yes, they're vegan), they can be enjoyed by vegans or strict vegetarians as well as everyone who likes meaty indulgences. The goal of this book is to provide you with inviting ways to eat more plants, period—no strings attached!

So, if you're following a plant-based or plant-forward (partly plant-based) lifestyle, you'll love these diabetes-friendly recipes to assist you on your health journey. If you're still a meat lover, I encourage you to simply sprinkle more plants into your meaty eating repertoire by slowly swapping these dishes into your current plan.

The appealing dishes (more than 125 of them!) in *The Plant-Based Diabetes Cookbook* are full of freshness, flavor, and real satisfaction. In fact, more than 50 of the recipes are main dishes.

Enjoyment is the only "rule" I have for the recipes! (Though I've kept the carbs in check so that you don't need to worry about easily going overboard.) All of the nutrition info is included for your reference, just in case you need it for your diabetes or overall health management, too.

The cooking directions are streamlined so that you don't need to follow dozens of steps to get your food to the table. And there's so much more for you to sink your teeth into in this book, including tips for following a plant-forward, diabetes-friendly lifestyle, strategies for punching up plant protein, and sample plant-based menus. Plus, you'll find a glossary at the end of this cookbook that includes select plant-based eating terms that may be new to you.

Whether you have diabetes, prediabetes, or just want to eat more plants, *The Plant-Based Diabetes Cookbook* will help bring nourishment to the table, deliciousness to your taste buds, and good health to your life. You'll appreciate having the flexibility so that you—or your diabetes care team—can plan meals to fit your personalized eating style and overall lifestyle. Cooking for others? Your family and friends will absolutely appreciate all of the benefits, too.

It's been such a treat to create these recipes for you.

Cheers to good health!

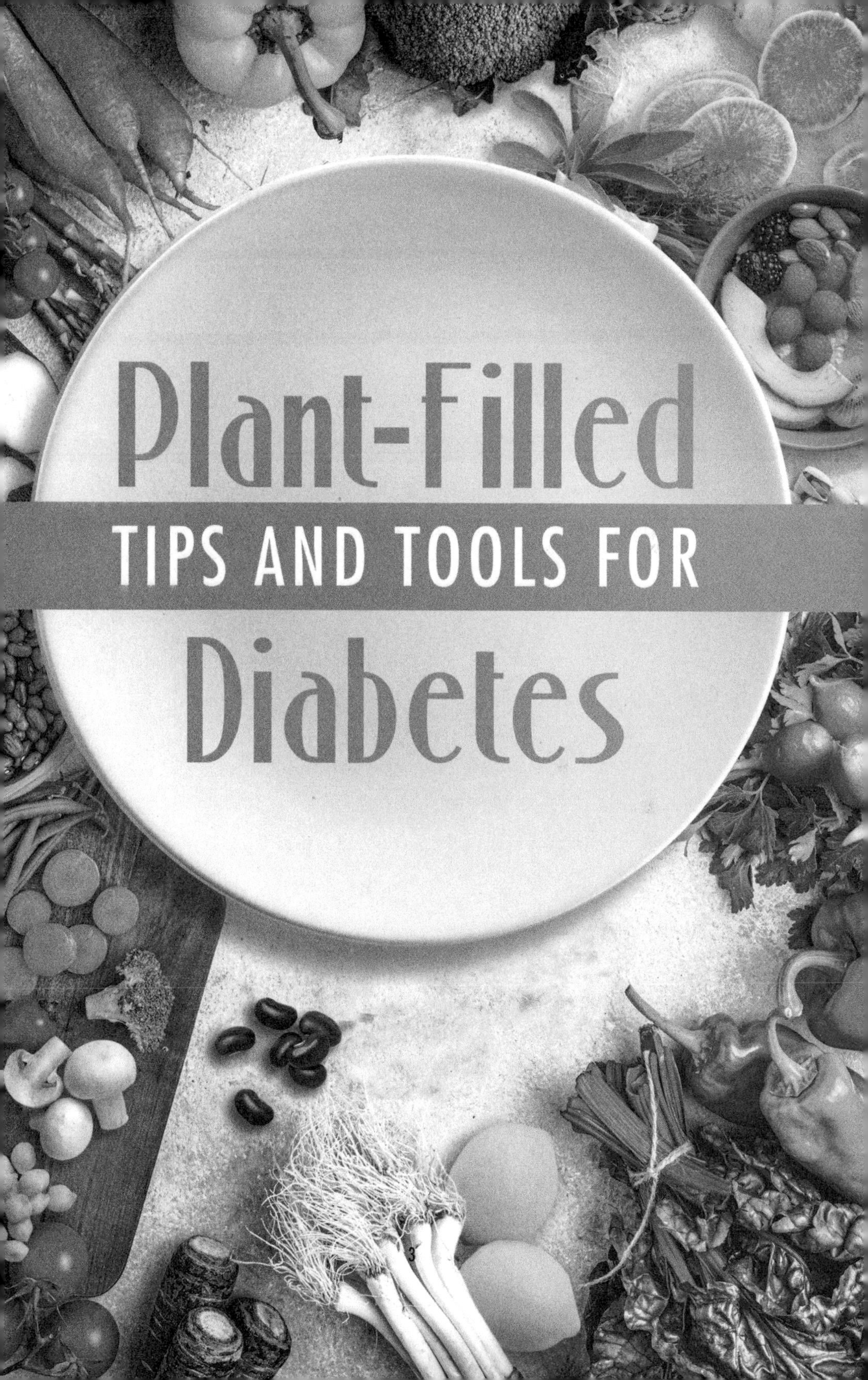
Plant-Filled
TIPS AND TOOLS FOR
Diabetes

Following a Plant-Forward, Diabetes-Friendly Lifestyle

Before diving into the scrumptiousness within the pages of this cookbook, I want to share some of the basics about diabetes, as a refresher, as well as information about how plant-based eating can fit into your diabetes eating plan. Don't worry, it's not overly science-y . . . just key highlights that everyone can understand.

I'll start with the not-so-good news. In the United States, diabetes is an epidemic with an estimated 130 million adults living with diabetes or prediabetes. Prediabetes means someone is at risk for developing type 2 diabetes. Here's a snapshot of what that means. In the US, more than one in ten people (11.3 percent) have diabetes, and nearly four in ten adults (38 percent) have prediabetes. Just looking at people sixty-five years or older, close to half (48.8 percent) have prediabetes. So, if you have diabetes or prediabetes, know that you're definitely not alone!

Now for the good news! Prediabetes does not need to become diabetes. And diabetes is fully manageable with proper treatment, ideally using a team approach, along with lifestyle changes. Instruction and counseling on nutrition therapy by a registered dietitian nutritionist (RDN) and/or a Certified Diabetes Care and Education Specialist (CDCES) can be especially beneficial.

Plus, following a high-quality, plant-based eating plan, while managing a healthy weight, may help curb diabetes. Research backs that up.

That's where this cookbook comes in handy. I developed all of the recipes in *The Plant-Based Diabetes Cookbook* with the needs of people with diabetes and prediabetes in mind. So you can absolutely feel good about what you're eating by including any of these dishes into your individualized eating plan.

What Is Diabetes?

It's good to know the facts. Diabetes is a chronic health condition. It means your body isn't able to turn the food you eat into energy as effectively as the bodies of those without diabetes. The result is high blood glucose levels, which can lead to damaged blood vessels in your heart, eyes, nerves, and kidneys.

The main forms of diabetes are type 1, type 2, and gestational diabetes. Type 2 diabetes is the most common form, affecting about 90–95 percent of those that have diabetes. Type 1 diabetes is a lifelong autoimmune disorder in which the pancreas doesn't make any insulin. During pregnancy, gestational diabetes can develop in women who don't have diabetes.

I have a family history of type 2, so I plan in diabetes-friendly recipes to try to prevent it! Eating and cooking right play essential roles in managing a healthy weight, which can be a vital strategy for managing type 2 diabetes. In fact, losing just a few pounds can help make diabetes management easier.

Are Carbs Bad?

The short answer is "no!" But the carbohydrates you eat do have a direct impact on your blood glucose. Therefore, it's helpful to spread out your carb intake throughout the day and try to steer clear of carb-rich meals. In other words, instead of 2 cups of pasta in a bowl, have 1 cup of pasta tossed with 1 or more cups of non-starchy veggies in that bowl. The goal isn't to go low carb; it's to eat the right amount of carbs for your body.

Your RDN, CDCES, or someone on your diabetes care team can help determine carbohydrate goals that are *right for you.* Know that being a strict "carb counter" is generally not required, though I find a helpful guide is to keep meals around 45 grams of total carbs (or less), unless you're highly active, in which case you'll want more.

What Foods Have Carbs?

Carbohydrates (or "carbs" for short) are a form of energy and are in much of our food supply! Your body breaks down carbs into glucose, which is the major fuel for your brain and muscles. Foods that contain significant carbs include vegetables, fruits, grains, dairy, beans, and also breads, pastas, sweets, and sodas. The carbohydrates in all of these foods affect your blood glucose levels, but some of these food choices are better for you than others. So focus on the quality of carbs you consume. Carbohydrate foods can be rich in fiber, vitamins, and minerals, *and* low in added sugars, saturated fats, and sodium.

It's beneficial for blood glucose management to aim mainly for carbohydrate-rich picks that are closest to nature (i.e., the least processed). For instance, choose mainly non-starchy vegetables, like salad greens, broccoli, cauliflower, asparagus, tomatoes, onions, and eggplant. And select mainly whole grains, like brown rice, farro, and freekeh (young green wheat), as well as whole-grain foods, like whole-wheat bread and whole-grain tortillas. As for fruit, enjoy it mainly whole rather than as juice. And, of course, try to choose "no-sugar-added" foods so that you can make the calories that you do get the most nourishing that they can be.

Selecting Your Plan

From here, it's mostly about personalization. You ideally want to follow a diabetes eating plan that fits your own preferences and goals. Yes, you definitely want a plan rather than no plan. I suggest keeping it as plant-based as possible for the most health benefits. Though that can also mean a plant-forward (or partly plant-based, "flexitarian," or semi-vegetarian) approach, especially if you're not ready to or prefer not to jump fully into 100 percent plant-based eating.

Whether you eat lots of plants or just more than you used to, using the American Diabetes Association's Diabetes Plate Method ("Create Your Plate") can be a helpful tool. Carbohydrate counting and special equipment is not required! For meals, the gist of this method is to fill half of your 9-inch plate with non-starchy veggies, a quarter with carb-rich foods (like starchy veggies, whole grains, or fruits), and a quarter with protein (yes, that can be plant protein, like black beans, nuts, and tofu). Add some healthy fats (such as avocado and extra-virgin olive oil) and zero calorie beverages to this, too. The same method can apply to mixed meals, such as stews, casseroles, or bowl meals. Pretty simple!

Going Plant-Based

Now you may be wondering just how plant-based you want to go. Ultimately, it's up to you, with guidance from your diabetes care team. But here's some info to help.

Following a plant-based eating pattern can have significant benefits for protecting your health. In fact, a review of the research suggests that when following a plant-based diet, people with type 2 diabetes were able to better manage their condition, including their HbA1c (more commonly known as A1C) levels, total cholesterol, and weight, as well as boost their mood and quality of life. Awesome, right?

In general, a plant-based eating plan or "diet" includes vegetables, fruits, whole grains, pulses, nuts, and seeds and excludes most or all animal products. Many people already eat more plant-based meals than they might realize. A peanut butter and jelly sandwich, spaghetti marinara, and a bean and veggie burrito can all be made vegan!

The bottom line: eating vegan (that is, 100 percent plant-based) meals offers the potential of improving parameters associated with type 2 diabetes.

Some people who follow a plant-based eating approach choose to eat dairy and eggs; research suggests that A1C levels can still be improved by following a vegetarian diet that includes both of these animal foods.

While you don't have to go fully plant-based or become a vegan (excluding all animal products from your diet and lifestyle), do plan to add some 100 percent plant-based meals to whatever your meal plan is. That'll be easy since every one of the recipes in *The Plant-Based Diabetes Cookbook* is completely plant-based.

What Are Other Benefits of Plant-Based Eating?

By eating mostly plants (foods grown thanks to Mother Earth!), you'll naturally be able to eat a significant amount of nutrients—including vitamins, minerals, antioxidants, fiber, and healthy (unsaturated) fats—which may play a protective role when you have diabetes. One special type of non-digestible fiber found in plants is *prebiotic fiber*; it feeds *probiotics* (the "good" bacteria in your gut) to potentially help protect your health. There may be a promising connection between having a healthy intestinal *microbiome* ("good" gut) and diabetes health.

Last, but not least, eating plant-based is associated with environmental sustainability, ultimately leading to a healthier planet! One reason for that is plant agriculture emits far less heat-trapping gasses, like carbon dioxide and methane, into the atmosphere than does animal agriculture. That means if you're trying to do your part to shrink your environmental footprint and curb our climate emergency, eating plant-based will have a beneficial impact.

Fortunately, *The Plant-Based Diabetes Cookbook* will help you incorporate as many fully plant-based meals into your eating repertoire as you wish. The fact that the recipes are so satisfying and delicious makes it a true pleasure.

Your Personal Checklist

Remember that the more personalized your meal plan is to your lifestyle, preferences, and diabetes health goals, the better. You are unique!

With that said, there are many nutrition-related tips that may be helpful for everyone with diabetes. I've created a doable list of some of the key strategies for managing diabetes. You can use it like an ongoing checklist. If you're newer to diabetes, simply pick three tips at a time. Once they become good habits, focus on three more. And know that this "shortcut" list doesn't replace routine visits with your diabetes care team.

- ✔ Check your blood glucose levels regularly.
- ✔ Know your A1C level.
- ✔ Stick to a regular eating schedule.
- ✔ Choose to chew, not drink, your calories most of the time.
- ✔ Go halfsies—filling half of your plate or bowl with non-starchy veggies.
- ✔ Choose whole grains instead of refined grains.
- ✔ Try fat swapping—opting for foods with healthier fats, like avocados, nuts, and olive oil.
- ✔ Aim for moderate sodium—ideally below 2,300 milligrams (mg) per day—not no sodium.*
- ✔ Do desserts wisely, occasionally, and with a plan.
- ✔ Pick "no-sugar-added" food and beverage options when you have the option.
- ✔ Move it (even just going for a long walk) regularly.
- ✔ Simply do the best you can!

**Hint: Sodium intake can be spread throughout the day. So, if one food or recipe you eat is high in sodium or simply seems overly salty, just balance it with lower sodium choices the rest of the day.*

A Well-Stocked, Plant-Based Pantry

Cooking diabetes-friendly, plant-based recipes isn't complicated. But if you don't have a properly stocked kitchen, it can seem a little challenging or time-consuming. So, stock up! It'll help to simplify the preparation of your meals and snacks from this cookbook and beyond.

Aim to have at least half of these ingredients on hand for a nutrient-rich pantry, fridge, and freezer. And remember to always practice "first in, first out"—also known as FIFO—to make sure you use the older ingredients first.

Kitchen Counter

- Non-starchy veggies, including grape tomatoes, onions, and garlic
- Fruits, including avocados and bananas
- Tea bags, including green or peppermint
- Black peppercorns (grind as needed)
- Sea salt

Pantry

- Nuts, including pistachios, pecans, walnuts, and peanuts*
- Seeds, including sunflower seeds, chia seeds, and pepitas*
- Nut and seed butters, including tahini

- Dried fruits, including dried unsulfured apricots, tart cherries, and raisins
- Whole grains, including oats, farro, quinoa (it's technically a seed), and brown rice
- Dry pulses, including lentils
- Pastas, pulse-based and whole-grain
- Low-sodium vegetable broth
- Canned tomatoes
- Canned beans, including black, pinto, red kidney, cannellini, and chickpeas (garbanzo beans)
- Heart-healthy oils, including avocado, sunflower, and extra-virgin olive
- Vinegars, including balsamic, red wine, and apple cider
- Soy sauce, naturally brewed, regular and/or reduced sodium
- Hot sauce
- Pure vanilla extract
- Dried herbs and spices (a variety!)
- Coconut sugar
- Nutritional yeast flakes

Fridge

- Non-starchy veggies, including eggplant, bell peppers, cauliflower, cucumber, broccoli, and zucchini
- Aromatics, including gingerroot, scallions, and hot chili peppers
- Berries, including strawberries, raspberries, and blueberries
- Lemons and limes and/or bottled lemon and lime juices (not from concentrate)
- Plant-based liquid eggs
- Plain, unsweetened, plant-based Greek-style yogurt
- Plain, unsweetened, plant-based milk
- Plant-based tree-nut cheese(s)
- Unsweetened applesauce
- Fruit-sweetened or no-sugar-added fruit spreads (jams)

- No-sugar-added ketchup, mustard, and barbecue sauce
- Vegan mayo
- Salsas
- Cheese-free pesto
- Tofu, soy-, chickpea- or pumpkin seed-based
- Tempeh
- Seitan
- Hummus

Freezer

- Frozen veggies, including petite peas and corn (it's technically a whole grain)
- Frozen pulses, including shelled edamame and lima beans
- Frozen fruits, including strawberries, raspberries, blueberries, and mango
- Frozen meat alternatives, including veggie burgers, plant-based chicken patties, and ground, plant-based meat

**Nuts and seeds can be refrigerated or frozen for longer storage.*

Tips to Punch Up Plant Protein

Whether you're following the recipes in this cookbook within your fully plant-based or plant-forward (partly plant-based) lifestyle, you'll want to get adequate protein in your eating plan. It's easy for meat eaters to just plop a steak onto their plate, pick up a chicken drumstick, or bite into a burger and get lots of protein. It takes just slightly more (but not much more) thought into getting this vital macronutrient in meatless meals.

Know that you can obtain all of the protein your body needs by eating 100 percent plant-based. Hey, if some professional athletes can do it, so can you!

First, know that protein is found naturally in significant amounts in most plant foods. While fruit is generally a low source of this macronutrient, you'll be able to get plenty of protein from beans, peas, chickpeas, lentils, nuts, seeds, whole grains, and vegetables. Protein is found in anything that's made with these foods too, like hummus, whole-grain bread, and marinara sauce. To make it easier, tofu, tempeh, and seitan are readily available—and the plant-based alternative food market is booming.

You'll also want to keep in mind that protein doesn't always have to be enjoyed in the form of an entrée. Besides a main dish, shift your concept of protein to something that you can obtain equally well in a side dish or appetizer, for instance.

Wherever and however you eat wholesome plant protein, it naturally offers *all* of the essential amino acids that your body needs. When you're fueling your body properly, you'll be getting all of those amino acids in the amounts that are important. Protein powders are not necessary for most people.

Try a taste of some of my personal favorite tips for punching up plant protein in your diabetes plant-based or plant-forward eating plan.

Seeds

Seeds used to get lost in the shadow of nuts, but they've powered their way to their own deserving place in the culinary spotlight.

- Pack a small snack pouch of shelled hemp seeds (hemp hearts) to go; they're ideal for sprinkling onto nearly anything when dining out.
- Use tahini (sesame seed paste) well beyond just in hummus, as in *Simple Lemony Tahini Sauce*—it's delicious drizzled over roasted veggies, in sandwiches, and more.
- Make chia gel to act as an egg replacer in your baking: Stir 1 tablespoon chia seeds with 3 tablespoons water (or other liquid) and swap for 1 egg.

ENJOY SEEDS IN THESE RECIPES: *Stuffed Veggie and Hummus Sandwich, Scrappy BBQ Bowl,* and *Maitake Gyro with Minty Tahini Sauce.*

Nuts

Eating about a handful of nuts regularly may help to reduce your risk of heart disease—and lucky for us they're so darn tasty.

- Make plant-based pesto; go heavy on nuts and use a duo, like pistachios and walnuts; sprinkle in nutritional yeast for zing; and pair with pulse-based pasta, roasted veggies, and more.
- To enhance nuttiness, pan-toast walnuts, pecans, pine nuts, and

natural sliced almonds in a dry skillet over medium-high before using them to finish a dish with bonus crunch.

- Don't forget about peanut butter—and almond butter, cashew butter, and pistachio butter. If a sandwich lover, don't forget about PB and J—and AB and J, CB and J, and the greener PB and J.

ENJOY NUTS IN THESE RECIPES: *Spicy Cashew Queso Dip, Tree-Nut Cheese, Grape and Pistachio Poppers,* and *Almond Cookie Balls.*

Pulses (Dry Beans, Peas, Chickpeas, and Lentils)

Canned beans are awesome! And so are the myriad culinary forms in which to get pulses, including pastas, flours, plant milks, yogurts, and snack foods.

- Sprinkle freshly roasted or packaged crispy roasted chickpeas, lentils, or fava beans onto salads or soups like they're croutons.
- Purée canned cannellini or great northern beans into vegetable-based soups or pasta sauces for velvety creaminess without the cream.
- Swap chickpea (garbanzo bean) or other pulse-based flour in place of half of the traditional flour in a recipe for baked goods, like quick breads, muffins, and cookies.

ENJOY PULSES IN THESE RECIPES: *Fluffy Pulse-Based Flatbread, Pulse Party Nachos,* and *French Lentil Salad.*

Organic Soybean Foods

I suggest choosing organic instead of traditional soybean foods since most of the soy grown in the US is genetically modified. Then enjoy soy in its various whole forms.

- Grill seasoned organic tofu slices, like *Blackened Orange and Ginger Tofu Filets,* just like it's steak. (Hint: Also try tofu made from chickpeas or pumpkin seeds instead of soybeans.)

- Sprinkle freshly prepared, shelled, organic edamame onto your morning avocado toast for nutrient balance and extra satisfaction.
- Make taco "meat" by sautéing crumbled organic tempeh and diced onion in oil for a few minutes, then simmering with taco seasoning and a big splash of veggie broth until absorbed.

ENJOY ORGANIC SOYBEAN FOODS IN THESE RECIPES: *Kung Pao Tofu and Peppers, Indian Sweet Potato Edamame Stew,* and *Barbecued Boneless Tempeh Ribs.*

Seitan

Seitan ("say-tan") is a wheat gluten food with a meaty texture (also known as "wheat meat") that's been around for eons. It's gotten new life today thanks to social media videos.

- Sauté unflavored seitan per package directions. Add chili powder, ground coriander, smoked paprika, cinnamon, and salt and pepper, and serve with toppings in a whole-grain pita as a gyro.
- Make sizzling fajitas using seitan as an ideal alternative to meat; simply season the seitan with ground cumin and chili powder and toss with salsa at the end of sautéing time.
- Create party-friendly skewers by preparing seitan, securing on skewers, brushing with a peanut sauce, like *Thai Peanut Dressing*, and serving with lime wedges.

ENJOY SEITAN IN THESE RECIPES: *Bell Pepper, Sweet Potato and "Sausage" Hash Skillet, Chorizo Seitan and Veggie Tacos*, and *Cajun Grain Mini-Bowl.*

Whole Grains

Aim to eat most of your grains as whole grains to obtain all edible grain parts—bran, germ, and endosperm (starchy layer). Choose oats, brown rice, farro, freekeh, teff, bulgur, and beyond.

- Pulse rolled oats in a food processor until they look like breadcrumbs, then use them in recipes as better-for-you breadcrumbs.

- To bulk up soup that's too brothy, stir in bulgur wheat and simmer for 10 minutes more.
- Add rinsed quinoa to a skillet over medium-low heat, and stir with a whisk until toasted. Sprinkle onto plant-based yogurt, salads, and vegan mac and cheese—or stir into melted dark chocolate to create a healthier chocolate crunch bar. (FYI: Botanically, quinoa is a seed.)

ENJOY WHOLE GRAINS IN THESE RECIPES: *Savory Herbed Mediterranean Oatmeal, Cajun Grain Mini-Bowl,* and *Dill Freekeh and Roasted Carrot Salad.*

Plant-Based Alternatives

Every popular animal-based food has a plant-based alternative. Though most are considered "processed," they taste more like their original counterparts and have become even more nutritious than in the past.

- Heat chick'n nuggets (vegan chicken nuggets) per package directions and toss onto a leafy salad for a kick of family-friendly protein. Try in a *Tahini Caesar-Style Salad Wrap with Crispy Chickpeas*, too.
- Sauté lots of broccoli and/or zucchini with garlic, toss with cooked, pulse-based pasta (and a little pasta water), and then with soft tree-nut cheese until an alfredo-style sauce forms.
- Prepare plant-based Italian sausage per package directions, then slice and stir into savory oatmeal made with veggie broth, tomatoes, spinach, and basil for a protein boost at breakfast.

ENJOY PLANT-BASED ALTERNATIVES IN THESE RECIPES: *Minty Kibbeh-Inspired "Meatballs," Chick'n and Zucchini Parmesan in a Pan,* and *Chilaquiles-Style Bowl.*

Fun Foods

Yes, plant-based food favorites can be a source of protein. Three "fun foods" (that's my name for them!) to embrace are cocoa powder, nutritional yeast, and avocados (one of the select fruits with a fair, but not high, amount of protein).

- Give cocoa powder life outside of dessert by exploring its savory side—try it like an earthy spice, especially in tomato-y sauces, chilis, and stews.
- Pop up a batch of popcorn (it's a whole grain!), then drizzle with extra-virgin olive oil and toss with nutritional yeast flakes, sea salt, black pepper, and fresh lemon zest. Yum!
- Make a savory whipped topping as a fluffy alternative to sour cream or guacamole; simply beat together avocado, vegan mayo, lemon juice, and salt, like *Avocado Crema.*

ENJOY FUN FOODS IN THESE RECIPES: *Fudgy Plant-Based Brownies, Squashed Chickpea "Eggs" with Plant-Based Goat Cheese,* and *Cool Avocado Soup.*

12 No-Recipe-Required Vegan Recipes

Not in a recipe-following mood? No problem! Make these no-brainer cuisine picks anytime you want a bite—big or small. Add your own tasty ideas and personalized variations to the list. When making shortcuts by purchasing store-bought, preprepped items, ideally choose preservative-free and no-sugar-added options for the most nourishment.

Apps and Snacks

Mediterranean Veggie Charcuterie Snack Board

On a wooden cutting board or small platter, arrange cherry tomatoes, cucumber slices, and bell pepper strips, along with ready-made hummus, a few olives, stuffed grape leaves, and wedges of whole-grain pita bread.

Grape, "Cheese," and Basil Skewers

Cut plant-based, fresh Italian-style mozzarella cheese into cubes; arrange on reusable skewers or bamboo picks with grapes or grape tomatoes and fresh basil leaves. Drizzle with balsamic vinegar reduction (glaze).

PB and J Plant-Based Yogurt Jar

Stir a few drops of pure vanilla extract into plain, unsweetened, plant-based Greek-style yogurt. Layer in a small jar with dollops of no-sugar-added peanut butter and fruit-sweetened strawberry fruit spread (jam). Sprinkle with roasted peanuts.

Grilled Figs and "Goat Cheese"

Halve fresh figs, lightly brush the cut sides with sunflower or avocado oil, and grill until grill marks form. Transfer to a plate and sprinkle with crumbled, plant-based, goat-style cheese, or dollops of soft tree-nut cheese of choice; then sprinkle with balsamic vinegar and fresh basil.

Main Dishes

Southwestern Big Bowl

Fill a big bowl with mixed salad greens. Arrange canned, drained red kidney or pinto beans, cooked veggie of choice (like roasted cauliflower), sliced avocado, grape tomatoes, and a few tortilla chips on the greens. Dress with salsa verde whisked with sunflower or avocado oil.

Green Hummus Flatbread Pizza

Grill or broil whole-grain flatbread or naan until toasted as desired. Blend hummus with several fresh spinach and/or basil leaves, then spread flatbread with the green hummus. Top with cucumber slices and pistachios, and sprinkle with extra-virgin olive oil and fresh parsley or basil leaves.

Cool Lentils

Toss canned, drained lentils with a generous amount of chopped fresh mint, parsley, and basil, minced scallions, quartered grape tomatoes, lemon vinaigrette (lemon juice whisked with extra-virgin olive oil), and a pinch of sea salt and black pepper. Sprinkle with soft tree-nut cheese of choice.

Pulse Pasta Pesto

Cook red lentil or chickpea pasta in boiling water per package directions; drain, toss with ice cubes to cool, and drain again. Toss with plant-based pesto sauce, lots of baby spinach, chopped pan-toasted walnuts, and some grated lemon zest and/or nutritional yeast flakes. Enjoy cool.

Jackfruit Tacos

Heat packaged, unseasoned, shredded jackfruit per package directions, stirring in salsa or salsa verde to flavor it. Stuff into whole-grain corn or grain-free tortillas with smashed black beans and shredded romaine. Top with dollops of guacamole.

Soup, Salad, and Side

Black Bean Soup

Combine equal parts canned and drained black beans, canned diced tomatoes with chilies, and low-sodium vegetable broth in a saucepan; simmer 10 minutes. Serve as is or blended, and top with plain, unsweetened, plant-based Greek-style yogurt, or vegan sour cream and chives.

Red and Green Salad

Attractively arrange large strips of freshly roasted red bell pepper or slices of vine-ripened tomato onto a salad plate and sprinkle with lemon vinaigrette (lemon juice whisked with extra-virgin olive oil), a pinch of sea salt, whole fresh mint leaves, and pan-toasted pine nuts.

Cajun Confetti Corn

Heat a little avocado oil in a skillet over medium-high heat; add equal parts diced red and green bell peppers and thawed frozen corn, and sauté until golden brown. Stir in thinly sliced scallions, a squirt of lime juice, a pinch of sea salt, and desired amount of salt-free Cajun seasoning.

Sample Plant-Based Menus

Having well-planned menus can be wise for helping you meet your diabetes goals. It can also be a timesaver because you know exactly what you need to shop for in advance. So here you go!

I love using the fun formula of *3 x 2 + 1*. This is how it works:

- Plan three days of meals and snacks for Sunday, Tuesday, and Thursday.
- Put them on repeat the next day, including "planned-overs" (intentional leftovers) so extra cooking isn't required for Monday, Wednesday, and Friday.
- Have one day (Saturday) to enjoy dining out, creatively eating leftovers, or crafting new meals using any extras.

You can change days as you like, such as starting menus on Monday, leaving Sunday as the extra day. Any which way you plan your menus, having three days of menus per week allows you to get plenty of variety without the extra time required for cooking. You can make anything in advance that you wish, too.

Here you'll find filling and flavorful menus to get you started. The *italicized* items are recipes in this cookbook. Go ahead and personalize the menus, adding any details you need, such as amounts. Then create your own menu based on this approach. Change your menus every week—or use the same ones for up to one month before switching them up. Swap in one of the *12 No-Recipe-Required Vegan Recipes* (pages 21–24) anytime you like. Serve all meals with calorie-free beverages, like water (of course!), flavored zero-calorie sparking water, or unsweetened green, black, or peppermint tea.

NOTE: *The sample menus below provide you with a general eating road map. Discuss with your registered dietitian nutritionist or certified diabetes care and education specialist if you need to follow a more structured eating plan.*

3 X 2 + 1 MENU ONE	SUNDAY + REPEAT DAY: MONDAY	TUESDAY + REPEAT DAY: WEDNESDAY	THURSDAY + REPEAT DAY: FRIDAY
BREAKFAST	*Cocoa-Covered Strawberry Overnight Oatmeal* (p. 81) Almonds	Fruit smoothie made with a protein-rich, unsweetened, plant-based milk, frozen sliced banana, chia seeds, and a few drops of pure vanilla extract Pistachios or walnuts	Plant-based scrambled eggs with fresh basil Pan-blistered cherry tomatoes Whole-grain toast drizzled with olive oil or spread with mashed avocado
LUNCH	Reduced-sodium vegan lentil soup topped with optional diced avocado Organic kale side salad tossed with sunflower oil, lemon juice, and sunflower seeds	*Tahini Caesar-Style Salad Wrap with Crispy Chickpeas* (p. 153) Falafel or veggie meatballs (or energy balls/bites)	Pasta salad made with pulse-based pasta, lots of non-starchy veggies (including broccoli and red onion), Italian vinaigrette, and plant-based "Parmesan" cheese

DINNER	Whole-grain tortilla stuffed with vegetarian refried beans, sautéed veggies (zucchini, bell peppers, baby bella mushrooms, and spinach), and pinch of vegan Mexican-style cheese, rolled up as a burrito, warmed in skillet, topped with *pico de gallo* or salsa	*Vegetable Mousse "Meatloaf"* (p. 117) Plant-based sour cream for "meat-loaf" topping Sautéed or roasted red bell pepper strips White beans served as salad splashed with lemon juice, olive oil, and basil	*Kung Pao Tofu and Peppers* (p. 91) Buckwheat soba noodles or brown rice Soy sauce with splash of rice vinegar
SNACKS (plan in one or two based on your needs)	*Wild Buffalo Chickpea Snackers* (p. 55) Black bean or other pulse-based dip with colorful bell pepper strips	Nut-based snack bar Guacamole with cherry tomatoes (stuff the tomatoes for fun)	Unsweetened plant-based Greek-style yogurt with blueberries *BBQ Stovetop Popcorn* (p. 57)

3 X 2 + 1 MENU TWO	SUNDAY + REPEAT DAY: MONDAY	TUESDAY + REPEAT DAY: WEDNESDAY	THURSDAY + REPEAT DAY: FRIDAY
BREAKFAST	*Avocado and Garbanzo Smash Toasts* (p. 73)	Unsweetened, plant-based yogurt bowl attractively topped with granola, pan-toasted sliced almonds, thawed frozen cherries, and chia seeds or cacao nibs	Savory oatmeal made with oats, low-sodium vegetable broth, spinach, and sliced sun-dried tomatoes, and topped with plant-based goat-style cheese and pumpkin seeds
LUNCH	Big bowl of mixed baby salad greens tossed with lemon juice and olive oil, generously topped with trail mix (nuts, seeds, and a little dried fruit)	*Saucy Peanut Soba Noodles with Slaw* (p. 167) Roasted peanuts to add to noodles	Frozen vegan entrée (350 to 400 calories) Pulse-based snack, such as crunchy roasted fava beans or lentils
DINNER	*Simple Spice-Rubbed Cauliflower Roast* (p. 97) Steamed edamame in pods with pinch of sea salt Mandarin orange	Bean- or lentil-based veggie burger in whole-grain English muffin with mustard and piled high with veggies Roasted green bean or carrot "fries"	*Chorizo Seitan and Veggie Tacos* (p. 143) Mixed berries or sliced apple Soft tree-nut cheese for taco topping or to pair with fruit

SNACKS (plan in one or two based on your needs)	Open-faced almond butter with fruit-sweetened raspberry jam on whole-grain toast Hummus with colorful bell pepper strips	*Nutty Candy Bar Minis* (p. 276) Grapes and wedge of aged vegan cheese	Raw veggie platter with plant-based tzatziki or baba ghanoush *Cool Avocado Soup* (p. 241) Pistachios and pomegranate arils for soup garnish

3 X 2 + 1 MY OWN MENU!	SUNDAY + REPEAT DAY: MONDAY	TUESDAY + REPEAT DAY: WEDNESDAY	THURSDAY + REPEAT DAY: FRIDAY
BREAKFAST			
LUNCH			
DINNER			
SNACKS (plan in one or two based on your needs)			

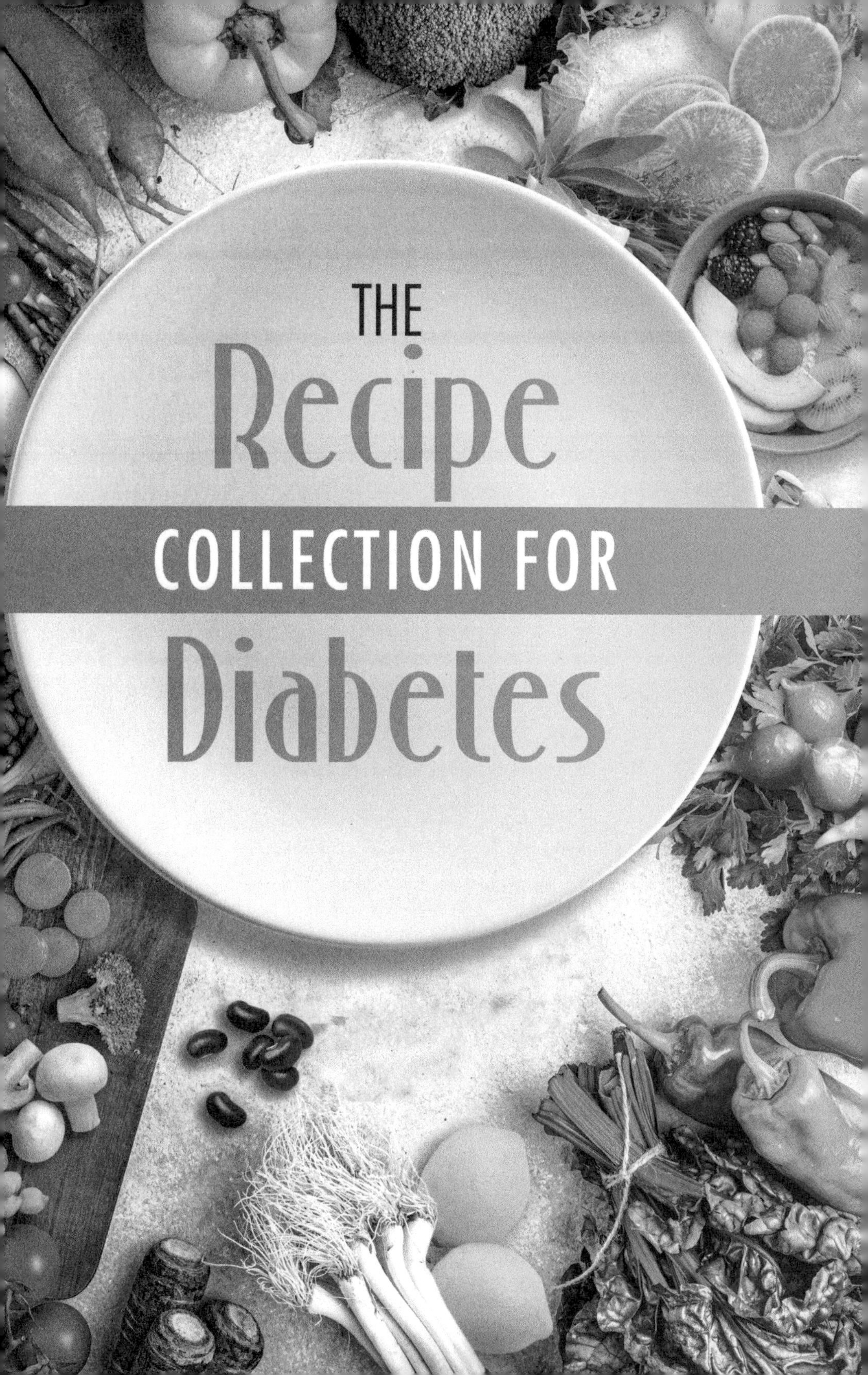
THE
Recipe
COLLECTION FOR
Diabetes

Party Apps and Snacks

AVOCADO CREMA

Have you tried avocado crema? It's a velvety topping based on avocados that's delightful on tacos and beyond. It kind of looks like fluffy green frosting! You'll adore how versatile it is as an alternative to guacamole, mayo, or sour cream. As a bonus, eating avocadoes is linked to a healthier overall dietary pattern and improved blood glucose regulation. So, try this creamy, nourishing, fully plant-based avocado crema soon—and often, like in *Breakfast Veggie Tacos* (page 65) and *Pulse Party Nachos* (page 61).

SERVES: 6 | SERVING SIZE: 2 tablespoons
PREP TIME: 8 minutes | COOK TIME: 0 minutes

- 1 fully-ripened avocado, pitted, quartered, and peeled
- 1 tablespoon vegan mayo or aquafaba "mayo"
- 1 teaspoon lemon or lime juice, or to taste
- ⅛ teaspoon sea salt, or to taste
- Pinch of cayenne pepper or chili powder (optional)

DIRECTIONS

In a mixer bowl, beat the avocado, vegan mayo, lemon juice, salt and, if using, cayenne until combined with an electric mixer on low speed. Then beat on high speed until velvety smooth and fluffy, at least 2 minutes.

NUTRITION INFO

Choices/Exchanges: 1 fat

Per serving: 45 calories, 4 g total fat, 0.5 g saturated fat, 0 g trans fat, 0 mg cholesterol, 65 mg sodium, 116 mg potassium, 2 g total carbohydrate, 2 g dietary fiber, 0 g sugars, 0 g added sugars, 0 g protein, 12 mg phosphorus

Mayonnaise Swaps

Classic mayonnaise is made with a vegetable oil, egg yolks, vinegar or lemon juice, salt, and sometimes a touch of mustard. But if you need a swap for it, like in this recipe, plant-based mayo-style products can be tasty alternatives. Vegan mayo (the term is abbreviated since it doesn't meet the traditional definition of "mayonnaise") can be made with various ingredients, such as a plant-based oil, like avocado oil, as well as water, vinegar, and/or lemon juice, salt, a little mustard oil or flour, and some plant protein. Another option is aquafaba "mayo," which features aquafaba—the intriguing liquid that remains from chickpea cooking or canning.

SPICY CASHEW QUESO DIP

If you're looking for a super creamy, highly flavored, cheesy-style dip, this is it! Luckily, it's got plenty of protein and is way better for you than a highly processed, nacho-cheese version that you may have indulged in as a teen. In fact, it's superfood-y. It's also speedy since you don't need to soak cashews—just use them as is. You can add more salsa to this recipe to adjust the taste to your palate. For not-so-spicy fans, simply use a mild salsa. No matter how spicy, it's delicious with tortilla chips, smeared over a veggie burger, or dolloped onto your *Plant-Based Bibb and Bean Burrito Bowl* (page 161) in place of the vegan cheese and salsa.

SERVES: 6 | SERVING SIZE: ¼ cup
PREP TIME: 15 minutes | COOK TIME: 0 minutes

- 5 ounces unsalted, unroasted cashews (1 cup)
- 1 garlic clove, chopped
- 2½ tablespoons nutritional yeast flakes
- ½ teaspoon chili powder
- ½ teaspoon ground paprika
- ½ teaspoon sea salt, or to taste
- ⅛ teaspoon ground turmeric
- ⅛ teaspoon freshly ground black pepper
- ⅔ cup hot unsweetened green tea or water, or as needed
- ¼ cup + 2 tablespoons "medium" or "hot" thick and chunky salsa, divided

DIRECTIONS

1. Add the cashews, garlic, nutritional yeast, chili powder, paprika, salt, turmeric, black pepper, tea, and ¼ cup of the salsa to a blender, cover, and purée on high speed until extra creamy, at least 3 minutes. For a thinner consistency, add more tea or water by the teaspoon.
2. Transfer the dip to a serving bowl, garnish with or swirl in the remaining 2 tablespoons salsa, and serve.

NUTRITION INFO

Choices/Exchanges: 1 high fat protein, ½ fat, ½ carbohydrate

Per serving: 150 calories, 11 g total fat, 2 g saturated fat, 0 g trans fat, 0 mg cholesterol, 210 mg sodium, 208 mg potassium, 9 g total carbohydrate, 2 g dietary fiber, 1 g sugars, 0 g added sugars, 6 g protein, 117 mg phosphorus

What Is Nooch?

A highlight of this recipe is nutritional yeast—popularly called nooch. It's an awesome source of vitamin B12, which is a vitamin found naturally in animal-based foods. That's one thing that makes "nooch" unique since it's not an animal source. If you're not familiar with the flavor of nutritional yeast, it's kind of like an earthy Parmesan cheese that kicks up taste. Frankly, I didn't care for it the first time I tried it, but now I'm completely hooked on this pantry staple.

Got Leftovers?

If you have any leftover dip, chill it in the fridge. Then before serving, gently reheat it in a saucepan with a drizzling of additional green tea or water.

FRESH FIG GUACAMOLE

Throughout the summer and fall, there are many delicious varieties of fresh figs to be found, such as Black Mission, Calimyrna, Tiger Stripe, and Kadota. Try different types in this out-of-the-ordinary guacamole recipe for extra enticement. The result is a definitively figgy, slightly spicy guacamole that's full of palate appeal. Dollop the chunky culinary joy onto Mexican-style dishes, like *Portabella "Steak" Fajitas* (page 87) or *No-Brainer Bean Burrito Wrap* (page 141), or simply scoop it up with blue corn tortillas or tortilla chips.

SERVES: 10 | SERVING SIZE: ¼ cup
PREP TIME: 12 minutes | COOK TIME: 0 minutes

- 2 Hass avocados, peeled, pitted, and cubed
- Juice of 1 lime (2 tablespoons)
- 3 fresh black mission figs, diced, or 2 dried figs, finely diced
- ¼ cup finely diced red onion
- 1 small jalapeño pepper with some seeds, minced
- 2 tablespoons finely chopped fresh cilantro
- 1 garlic clove, minced (optional)
- ½ teaspoon sea salt
- ⅛ teaspoon ground coriander
- ⅛ teaspoon ground cumin (optional)

DIRECTIONS

Gently stir together all ingredients in a medium bowl until just combined and serve.

NUTRITION INFO

Choices/Exchanges: 1 fat

Per serving: 50 calories, 3.5 g total fat, 0 g saturated fat, 0 g trans fat, 0 mg cholesterol, 100 mg sodium, 155 mg potassium, 5 g total carbohydrate, 2 g dietary fiber, 2 g sugars, 0 g added sugars, 1 g protein, 15 mg phosphorus

You Go, Grill

Having a cookout? If you've got your grill going, then take this *Fresh Fig Guacamole* to the next level. Halve the fresh figs, extra-lightly brush the cut surfaces with avocado or sunflower oil, grill until rich grill marks form, and then dice before adding to this guacamole. The grilled fig version is especially divine thanks to the aromatic hint of smokiness.

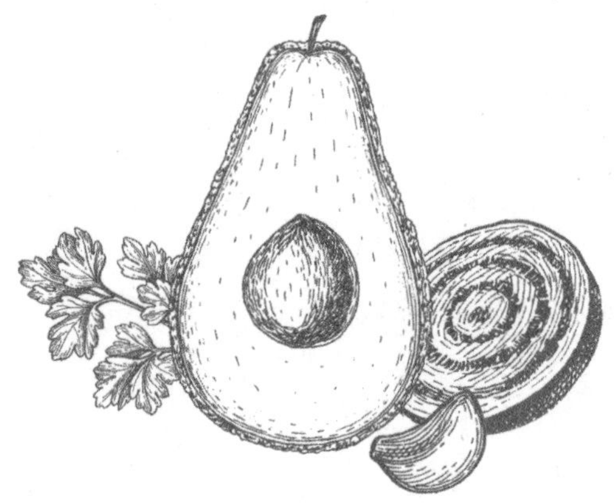

TREE-NUT CHEESE, GRAPE, AND PISTACHIO POPPERS

Not only are these poppers fun to eat, they're awesomely nutritious. They're simply grapes, covered in soft tree-nut cheese, and rolled in a crunchy pistachio mixture that you pop into your mouth as an appetizer, snack, or party hors d'oeuvre. If you want to be fancy, call them truffles. If you want to be playful, serve these as pops by inserting an appetizer-size bamboo pick into each popper. And if you want to go desserty, use this same recipe; swap about 8 to 10 strawberries in place of the grapes; and instead of black pepper, add a pinch of cinnamon. The taste is a little reminiscent of strawberry cheesecake!

SERVES: 10 | SERVING SIZE: 2 poppers (truffles)
PREP TIME: 20 minutes (including freezing time) | COOK TIME: 0 minutes

- 20 medium or 16 extra-large red seedless grapes
- 6 ounces plain, plant-based goat-style cheese or other soft spreadable-style tree-nut cheese
- 1 cup chopped, lightly salted, roasted pistachios (6.6 ounces)
- 1 teaspoon grated lemon zest
- ½ teaspoon freshly ground black pepper

DIRECTIONS

1. Wash and fully dry the grapes. One by one, form the plant-based goat-style cheese around each grape using your (clean!) hands. Then freeze for 5 minutes to slightly firm up.
2. In a small bowl, stir together the pistachios, lemon zest, and pepper. Firmly roll each "cheese" ball in the pistachio mixture to fully coat.
3. Keep cool until ready to serve. Serve like truffles.

NUTRITION INFO

Choices/Exchanges: 1 high fat protein, 1 fat, ½ fruit

Per serving: 170 calories, 12 g total fat, 1.5 g saturated fat, 0 g trans fat, 0 mg cholesterol, 95 mg sodium, 263 mg potassium, 10 g total carbohydrate, 2 g dietary fiber, 3 g sugars, 0 g added sugars, 6 g protein, 155 mg phosphorus

Go Nuts for Your Heart

Regularly eating nuts may play a role in reducing the risk of cardiovascular disease for people with type 2 diabetes. Choose a variety, such as pistachios, walnuts, almonds, cashews, pecans, and pine nuts. Buy lots and stash them in jars or silicone storage pouches in your freezer. Keep some in your pantry or on your kitchen countertop too so you can easily sprinkle onto salads or entrées, or use in recipes like this, for bonus crunch and enjoyment anytime. And yes, eating nut "cheese" can count as a heart-friendly pick, too!

MINTY KIBBEH-INSPIRED "MEATBALLS"

A popular Middle Eastern meat and bulgur wheat dish is called kibbeh. As a kid, I enjoyed it often—even in its raw form! I guess that's what happens when you're raised by a Lebanese mom. But this recipe is just loosely inspired by classic kibbeh. It's based on plant-based "meat" (I use Beyond Meat here) and changed a bit more to create a simple, flavorful fix. No, it's not raw! Enjoy these "meatballs" as a finger food as is, serve on a lemony leafy salad, or glam them up as you wish.

SERVES: 4 | SERVING SIZE: 3 "meatballs"
PREP TIME: 15 minutes | COOK TIME: 11 minutes

- ½ medium red or white onion, cut into 4 wedges
- ⅓ cup old-fashioned, whole-grain, rolled oats
- ¼ cup packed fresh mint leaves
- ¾ teaspoon ground cinnamon
- ½ teaspoon ground cumin
- ½ teaspoon garlic powder
- ½ teaspoon freshly ground black pepper
- ¼ teaspoon + ⅛ teaspoon sea salt
- 8 ounces uncooked, non-GMO, plant-based ground "meat"

DIRECTIONS

1. Preheat the oven to 475°F. Line a large, rimmed baking sheet with a silicone baking mat or unbleached parchment paper.
2. Add the onion to a food processor and blend until finely grated. Add the oats and mint and blend until finely chopped. Add the cinnamon, cumin, garlic powder, pepper, and salt and blend until evenly combined and a textured dough-like mixture forms. (Hint: Scrape down the insides of the food processor container as needed throughout this step.)
3. Transfer the mixture to a medium bowl, add the plant-based "meat," and stir until well combined. Form by hand or with a cookie scoop into 12 meatballs, about 2 tablespoons mixture each, and arrange on the baking sheet.
4. Roast in the oven for 6 minutes; flip over each meatball; and roast until well done and browned, about 5 minutes more. Serve the "meatballs" warm with small bamboo picks or toothpicks.

NUTRITION INFO

Choices/Exchanges: ½ carbohydrate, 2 lean protein, 1 fat

Per serving: 170 calories, 10 g total fat, 2.5 g saturated fat, 0 g trans fat, 0 mg cholesterol, 400 mg sodium, 202 mg potassium, 9 g total carbohydrate, 2 g dietary fiber, 1 g sugars, 0 g added sugars, 11 g protein, 31 mg phosphorus

Go Glam or Go Big

For wow-worthiness, serve these "meatballs" on a "bed" of plain, unsweetened, plant-based yogurt (try a chickpea- or tree-nut-based one), hummus, or baba ghanoush, then sprinkle with extra-virgin olive oil, pomegranate arils, and small fresh mint leaves. Or transform this recipe into grilled Middle Eastern–style "burgers." Serve in whole-grain pita along with lettuce, tomato, cucumber, and a tahini sauce—or use leafy greens as your bun for a carb-friendly fix.

Plant-Based Ground "Meat"

I love using lentils and finely chopped mushrooms as plant-based alternatives to ground meat. However, occasionally going for convenience by using a brand like Beyond Meat can be fine; just make sure it's based on non-GMO plant ingredients so that it's an environmentally conscious choice. And plan to pair it with veggies or whole grains or both—mixed in or added on—to enhance wholesomeness.

BALSAMIC ROASTED BRUSSELS SPROUTS SKEWERS

Serving on skewers adds a fun factor to cuisine. But often when a food is served on skewers, it's likely something meaty, like chicken satay, beef brochette, or shish kebab. You can change that with these hearty 100 percent vegetable kebabs. This secretly simple recipe will make a truly memorable bite—even for meat lovers. For an extra pop of party worthiness, arrange the brussels sprouts skewers on a serving platter and sprinkle with pomegranate arils (seeds).

SERVES: 8 I SERVING SIZE: 1 skewer
PREP TIME: 15 minutes I COOK TIME: 22–25 minutes

- 1½ pounds medium brussels sprouts (about 32 sprouts), trimmed, and halved lengthwise
- 2½ tablespoons extra-virgin olive oil, divided
- 1 teaspoon aged balsamic or pomegranate vinegar
- ¾ teaspoon freshly ground black pepper
- ½ teaspoon sea salt
- 2 tablespoons pomegranate arils (optional)

DIRECTIONS

1. Preheat the oven to 425°F. In a large bowl, toss together the halved brussels sprouts, 2 tablespoons of the oil, the vinegar, pepper, and salt. Transfer to a large rimmed baking sheet and arrange in a single layer, cut side up.
2. Roast until well caramelized and just tender on the inside, about 22–25 minutes, flipping over sprout halves halfway through the roasting process. Let stand about 5 minutes to complete the cooking process
3. Thread sprout halves onto 8 (8-inch) skewers, about 8 sprout halves each. Brush or drizzle with the remaining ½ tablespoon oil.
4. Transfer to a serving platter and, if desired, sprinkle with the pomegranate arils. Serve immediately or keep warm in a 200°F oven until ready to serve.

NUTRITION INFO

Choices/Exchanges: 1 vegetable, 1 fat

Per serving: 70 calories, 4.5 g total fat, 0.5 g saturated fat, 0 g trans fat, 0 mg cholesterol, 160 mg sodium, 300 mg potassium, 7 g total carbohydrate, 7 g dietary fiber, 2 g sugars, 0 g added sugars, 3 g protein, 55 mg phosphorus

Sizing Trick

When the fresh brussels sprouts you use vary significantly in size, it can mean some will get overcooked while others a bit undercooked during roasting. So, try this. Place the large sprouts on the left side of the baking sheet and the smaller ones on the right side. Remove the smaller ones from the oven a few minutes before the larger ones.

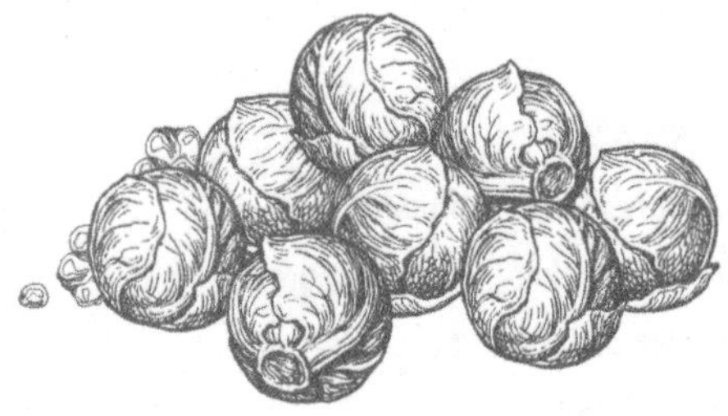

PAN-GRILLED SESAME TOFU SKEWERS

If you're looking for an introduction or reintroduction to tofu, say "hello" to these Szechwan skewers. They offer a truly tasty way to try tofu for the first time, or the umpteenth time! Marinated in a fresh gingery vinaigrette, inserted onto skewers, grilled until rich grill markings form, and garnished with fresh cilantro leaves and sesame seeds, these tofu "pops" are sure to be a hit for all the senses. Try them at your next cook-in . . . or cookout!

SERVES: 6 | SERVING SIZE: 3 skewers
PREP TIME: 20 minutes (plus marinating time) | COOK TIME: 8 minutes

- 2 tablespoons naturally brewed soy sauce
- 1½ tablespoons rice or brown rice vinegar
- 1 scallion, green and white parts, minced
- 1 tablespoon freshly grated gingerroot
- 1 tablespoon unsweetened applesauce
- 2 teaspoons toasted sesame oil
- ¼ teaspoon dried hot pepper flakes
- 1 (14-ounce) package extra-firm organic tofu*, drained and squeezed of excess liquid
- 1 teaspoon black or white sesame seeds (or a mixture), pan-toasted
- 2 tablespoons fresh small cilantro leaves

**Note: Use tofu that's made from soybeans (traditional), chickpeas, or pumpkin seeds.*

DIRECTIONS

1. Whisk together the soy sauce, vinegar, scallion, ginger, applesauce, sesame oil, and hot pepper flakes in a small bowl. (Makes ½ cup.) Pour into a 9- by 13-inch dish or similar-sized pan.
2. Cut the tofu lengthwise into 9 slices; then cut each slice in half lengthwise or crosswise, creating 18 pieces. Place the tofu slices in a single layer in the soy sauce mixture and marinate about 10 to 15 minutes per side.
3. Preheat a grill pan over medium-high heat. Transfer tofu slices to a platter or rimmed plate using tongs, reserving the marinade. Grill in batches until deep grill marks form on both sides, about 3½ to 4 minutes per side.

4. Insert reusable or bamboo skewers into the cooked tofu, sprinkle with the sesame seeds and cilantro leaves, and serve while warm with the remaining marinade on the side.

NUTRITION INFO
Choices/Exchanges: 1 medium fat protein
Per serving: 90 calories, 6 g total fat, 0.5 g saturated fat, 0 g trans fat, 0 mg cholesterol, 310 mg sodium, 100 mg potassium, 3 g total carbohydrate, 1 g dietary fiber, 1 g sugars, 0 g added sugars, 7 g protein, 90 mg phosphorus

Tofu and Diabetes

Wondering if you should be eating tofu (or more of it)? If you have type 2 diabetes, prediabetes, or are at risk for diabetes, the answer is yes! Studies suggest that eating (traditional soy based) tofu may be linked to a reduced risk of type 2 diabetes. Plant-based compounds called soy isoflavones seem to have anti-diabetic properties!

PLANT-BASED FETA AND PESTO QUESADILLAS

You're probably thinking either that quesadillas couldn't possibly be good for you or that, if they are, they certainly wouldn't taste very good. Right? Well, I hope to prove you wrong with these sort-of-Mexican, sort-of-Greek quesadillas—a really unique flavor combination. You'll whirl up a fresh and simple plant-based pesto that you'll slather into the tortillas. And hummus makes the filling desirably creamy. These quesadillas are bursting with international flavor.

SERVES: 6 | SERVING SIZE: 2 wedges
PREP TIME: 15 minutes | COOK TIME: 12 minutes

- ½ cup packed, fresh basil leaves
- Juice of ½ lemon (about 1½ tablespoons)
- 2 tablespoons pine nuts or chopped walnuts
- 2 teaspoons extra-virgin olive oil
- ¼ teaspoon sea salt
- ¼ teaspoon freshly ground black pepper
- 6 (8-inch) whole-grain or grain-free flour tortillas
- Organic oil cooking spray
- ⅓ cup finely crumbled, plant-based feta-style cheese*
- 1 cup packed, chopped, fresh baby spinach
- 2 scallions, green parts only, minced
- 3 tablespoons hummus of choice (see recipes in this book)

**Note: Ideally, choose vegan cheese products based on tree nuts.*

DIRECTIONS

1. Place the basil, lemon juice, pine nuts, oil, salt, and pepper into a food processor and pulse until the mixture has a pesto-like consistency.
2. Lay the tortillas on a large baking sheet and lightly coat with cooking spray (or extra-lightly brush with sunflower or avocado oil). Flip the tortillas over, sprayed side down. Spread the basil pesto over the entire surface of three of these tortillas and then sprinkle with the plant-based cheese, spinach, and scallions.

3. Spread the remaining three tortillas with the hummus and place onto the spinach-topped tortillas, hummus side down. Firmly press each quesadilla with a spatula to compact the ingredients.
4. Heat a large stick-resistant skillet over medium-high heat. Cook the quesadillas in batches until toasted, about 2 minutes per side. Cut each quesadilla into 4 wedges and serve warm.

NUTRITION INFO
Choices/Exchanges: 1 starch, ½ carbohydrate, 1½ fat
Per serving: 170 calories, 7 g total fat, 3.5 g saturated fat, 0 g trans fat, 0 mg cholesterol, 400 mg sodium, 147 mg potassium, 22 g total carbohydrate, 3 g dietary fiber, 2 g sugars, 0 g added sugars, 4 g protein, 18 mg phosphorus

Types of Tortillas

The choice used to just be between white or wheat flour tortillas or corn tortillas. And sometimes between soft or hard shell. But the variety of tortilla types available in the market today is expansive, with an array of exciting alternatives. Personally, I'm a sprouted whole-grain fan. Also be on the lookout for cauliflower, almond, sweet potato, cactus, coconut, and cassava, chickpea, and quinoa flour tortillas. One of the lower-carb, grain-free options may fit best into your diabetes eating plan. See the labels—and be enticed!

EDAMAME DUMPLINGS

Edamame—which is actually an immature soybean—has a cute name, lovely green color, exceptional nutritiousness, and lots of appeal. But many people still just order it as a sharable appetizer at a restaurant instead of enjoying it in culinary delights at home. So, here's one for you. The edamame is puréed with high-flavored ingredients, including hoisin sauce, and combined with aromatics, including fresh gingerroot, to create a memorable dumpling filling. Enjoy the dumplings simply as is or pair them with a dipping sauce, such as Gochujang, soy sauce, or a mixture of the two.

SERVES: 8 | serving size: 3 dumplings
PREP TIME: 25 minutes | cook time: 30 minutes

- 1½ cups frozen, shelled, organic edamame (7 ounces)
- 1 tablespoon hoisin sauce
- 2 teaspoons toasted sesame oil
- 1½ teaspoons naturally brewed soy sauce
- ¼ teaspoon dried hot pepper flakes
- 3 scallions, green and white parts, minced
- 2 teaspoons freshly grated gingerroot
- 1 large garlic clove, minced
- 1 tablespoon finely chopped fresh cilantro
- 24 round, plant-based dumpling wrappers
- Organic oil cooking spray

DIRECTIONS

1. Boil the edamame according to package directions. Drain, rinse with cold water (or toss with ice cubes to cool), and drain again. Add the edamame, hoisin sauce, sesame oil, soy sauce, and hot pepper flakes to a food processor. Cover and blend until the mixture forms a thick, smooth paste, scraping down the sides as needed. Transfer to a medium bowl and stir in the scallions, ginger, garlic, and cilantro until combined.
2. Keep the dumplings covered with a clean, damp kitchen towel. One at a time, brush the edges of each wrapper with fresh cold water. Place 2 teaspoons of the edamame mixture in the center of the wrapper. Fold one side of the wrapper over the filling to form into a half moon and pinch the edges. Crimp the edges with fork tongs, if desired.

3. Preheat the oven to 200°F. In a large saucepan, bring about 1 inch of water to a simmer over medium heat. Spritz a steamer basket with cooking spray (or extra-lightly brush with avocado oil or sunflower oil) to help prevent sticking before each batch. Place 8 of the dumplings (or as many dumplings as can fit) into the steamer without touching.
4. Cover and steam until the dumplings are cooked through, about 10 minutes. Remove the dumplings from the steamer to a heatproof platter and place in the oven to keep warm. (Spritz the dumplings with cooking spray, if necessary, to prevent sticking and keep moist.) Repeat until all of the dumplings are steamed, adding additional water for simmering between batches, if necessary.
5. Transfer the dumplings to a platter or individual plates and garnish with additional minced scallions (green parts), if desired. Enjoy the dumplings while warm.

NUTRITION INFO
Choices/Exchanges: 1 starch
Per serving: 80 calories, 2.5 g total fat, 0 g saturated fat, 0 g trans fat, 0 mg cholesterol, 140 mg sodium, 160 mg potassium, 12 g total carbohydrate, 1 g dietary fiber, 2 g sugars, 0 g added sugars, 4 g protein, 60 mg phosphorus

LEMONY WHITE BEAN AND ROSEMARY CROSTINI

This lovely crostini with its fragrant, velvety bean topping on crisp toasted baguette is downright sexy. It's so satisfying with its trio of fiber, healthy fats, and plant protein, too. It works equally well served as a party app or as a snack. To enjoy at snack time, stash the cannellini bean purée in the fridge; toast the bread slices and store in a sealed food container at room temperature; then make each serving as you like over the next three or four days. Or skip the baguette and make just the citrusy bean topping to enjoy as a divine dip all on its own. Serve it just like hummus or try it on a sandwich as a great-for-you condiment.

SERVES: 8 | SERVING SIZE: 3 crostini
PREP TIME: 12 minutes | COOK TIME: 1 minute

- 1 (15-ounce) can cannellini or other white beans, well-drained
- 3 garlic cloves, halved, divided
- Juice and zest of 1 small lemon (about 2 tablespoons juice)
- 1 tablespoon extra-virgin olive oil, or as needed
- ½ teaspoon finely chopped fresh rosemary leaves
- ¼ teaspoon sea salt
- 1 (6-ounce) whole-grain baguette, cut into 24 slices, removing bread ends*

**Note: Ideally, the slices will be about ½-inch thick from a traditional French baguette.*

DIRECTIONS

1. Preheat the broiler. Purée the beans, 2 of the garlic halves, lemon juice, oil, rosemary, and salt in a blender until smooth. If necessary, add 1-2 tablespoons cold water until the bean mixture reaches desired consistency. (Be patient with the blending process, scraping down sides as needed. The thicker the bean purée, the better.) Chill until ready to serve.
2. Broil the baguette slices until toasted, about 20-30 seconds per side. Once toasted, immediately rub the bread pieces with the cut end of the remaining garlic clove halves.

3. Just before serving, dollop (don't spread) the bean purée on top of each slice. If desired, drizzle with additional olive oil or garnish with additional rosemary leaves. Top with lemon zest. Serve at room temperature.

NUTRITION INFO

Choices/Exchanges 1 starch, 1 fat

Per serving: 120 calories, 3 g total fat, 0 g saturated fat, 0 g trans fat, 0 mg cholesterol, 250 mg sodium, 210 mg potassium, 18 g total carbohydrate, 4 g dietary fiber, 1 g sugars, 0 g added sugars, 6 g protein, 115 mg phosphorus

Buy BPA-Free

When buying canned beans, be sure to choose those with BPA-free lined cans. Luckily, the vast majority of canned foods manufactured in the US now use alternative liners that are free of BPA. However, it's still important to know what it is. BPA is a chemical whose longer name is Bisphenol A. Some scientists suggest that it may disrupt regular hormone activity in the body. You can check bean company websites or contact their customer service for specific information about their products.

HERB AND SPICE "EGG" SALAD BRUSCHETTA

If you're a fan of egg salad, you'll be enthused about this fully plant-based twist on it. It really does look like egg salad. But don't think of it as a substitute; it's an appetizing, protein-packed star all on its own. The spices of the tofu-based salad create notable kick and the herbs provide springy aroma. It's awesome served as bruschetta. They're not glamorous, just good grub. I use light rye crispbread to provide great crunch and satisfaction and keep this calorie conscious. Most importantly to everyone's taste buds, this bruschetta is delightfully delish.

SERVES: 6 I SERVING SIZE: 2 bruschetta
PREP TIME: 20 minutes (plus 1 hour chilling time) I COOK TIME: 0 minutes

- 2 scallions, green and white parts, minced
- 3 tablespoons vegan mayo or aquafaba "mayo"
- 1½ tablespoons whole-grain mustard
- 1½ tablespoons finely chopped, fresh flat-leaf parsley
- 1 tablespoon finely chopped, fresh tarragon
- ¼ teaspoon ground cayenne pepper, or to taste
- ¼ teaspoon ground turmeric
- ¼ teaspoon + ⅛ teaspoon sea salt, or to taste
- ¼ teaspoon freshly ground black pepper, or to taste
- 1 medium stalk celery, finely diced
- 1 (14-ounce) package firm organic tofu,* drained and squeezed of excess liquid
- 12 slices light rye or seeded crispbread

**Note: Use tofu that's made from soybeans (traditional), chickpeas, or pumpkin seeds.*

DIRECTIONS

1. Stir together the scallions, mayo, mustard, parsley, tarragon, cayenne, turmeric, salt and pepper in a medium bowl until well-combined. Add the celery and stir until evenly combined.
2. Mash the tofu in a large bowl using a large spoon until small, bite-sized crumbles are formed.

3. Stir the tofu into the celery mixture. Chill for at least 1 hour to let flavors blend. Adjust seasoning.
4. Top each crispbread with about 3 tablespoons of the tofu mixture and serve.

NUTRITION INFO

Choices/Exchanges: 1 starch, 1 lean protein, 1 fat

Per serving: 170 calories, 9 g total fat, 1.5 g saturated fat, 0 g trans fat, 0 mg cholesterol, 360 mg sodium, 200 mg potassium, 16 g total carbohydrate, 4 g dietary fiber, 1 g sugars, 0 g added sugars, 7 g protein, 130 mg phosphorus

Crispbread Alternatives

While this cool bruschetta recipe is crafted to use crispbread, you can serve the "egg" salad using other delicious "delivery vehicles." Stuff the salad in or on avocado or tomato halves, celery stalks, lettuce boats, seeded crackers, or grain-free wraps. Or go off course a bit and enjoy in a *Portabella BLT Sandwich with Heirloom Tomatoes* (page 151) or as a salad topper.

WILD BUFFALO CHICKPEA SNACKERS

I've got a serious crush on chickpeas! How about you? For all of us with a culinary fondness for the popular beans, this oven-roasted recipe offers a way to enjoy them as an anytime snack. They're also surprisingly versatile and lovable as garnishes or salad toppers, like in *Party Hummus Canapes* (page 59) or *Tahini Caesar-Style Salad Wrap with Crispy Chickpeas* (page 153). And while they don't actually taste like wild buffalo chicken wings, their flavor is inspired by that party-friendly food. Your taste buds will get a kick out of 'em.

SERVES: 4 | SERVING SIZE: 1/3 cup
PREP TIME: 5 minutes | COOK TIME: 25 minutes

- 1 (15-ounce) can no-salt-added garbanzo beans (chickpeas), well-drained
- 1 tablespoon extra-virgin olive oil
- 2 teaspoons hot pepper sauce, or to taste
- 2 teaspoons white wine vinegar
- ¼ teaspoon sea salt, or to taste
- 1½ teaspoons nutritional yeast flakes (optional)

DIRECTIONS

1. Preheat the oven to 425°F. Line a large rimmed baking sheet with a silicone baking mat or unbleached parchment paper.
2. Add the beans and oil to a medium bowl; toss to combine. Add the hot pepper sauce, white wine vinegar, and salt; toss to combine.
3. Arrange the beans in a single layer on the baking sheet. Bake until the beans are crisp on the outside and still creamy in the center, about 25 minutes. If desired, sprinkle with the nutritional yeast flakes.
4. Serve while warm or at room temperature. (Hint: They're best when enjoyed immediately while crisp.)

NUTRITION INFO
Choices/Exchanges: 1 starch, 1 lean protein, ½ fat
Per serving: 150 calories, 5 g total fat, 0.7 g saturated fat, 0 g trans fat, 0 mg cholesterol, 240 mg sodium, 210 mg potassium, 19 g total carbohydrate, 5 g dietary fiber, 3 g sugars, 0 g added sugars, 6 g protein, 120 mg phosphorus

No Rinsing Required!

There's no need to rinse beans when choosing a no-salt added variety. But if you prefer rinsing them, go for it. For best results, ensure that they're well-drained by wrapping the beans in a clean kitchen towel before use in this recipe.

What's a Silicone Baking Mat?

You'll notice several of my recipes suggest using a silicone baking mat-lined baking sheet. It's a reusable mat that's made from food-grade silicone. It offers a great way to help make the baking surface a smooth, nonstick one without the need for additional calories. It can stand up to high temperatures and helps with even heat distribution. It makes clean-up easy and, since reusable, there's no waste.

Hint: A silicone baking mat can also be used for kitchen prep, like rolling out pizza dough.

BBQ STOVETOP POPCORN

Is popcorn a "junk" food? Absolutely not! It's a whole-grain food. Though, if you mindlessly eat an oversized bucketful of the movie-friendly munchie, served heavily salted and doused in ladles of butter or a strange, butter-like substance as it's served at some theaters, then it actually does become a little "junky." This recipe is definitely not that. First, I suggest starting with USDA organic-certified popcorn, which means it'll be non-GMO. Then you'll pop it in heart-friendly oil and kick up its flavor with smoky paprika, BBQ sauce, and "nooch." Pop a batch for movie night—or any night—soon, and embrace popcorn's whole-grain goodness.

SERVES: 2 | SERVING SIZE: 2½ cups
PREP TIME: 5 minutes | COOK TIME: 10 minutes

- 1 tablespoon no-sugar-added barbecue sauce or *Fruit-Sweetened BBQ Sauce* (recipe follows)
- ½ teaspoon smoked paprika
- 1/8 teaspoon sea salt
- 1 tablespoon avocado oil or sunflower oil
- ¼ cup unpopped popcorn kernels
- 1½ teaspoons nutritional yeast flakes (aka "nooch")

Directions

1. In a small bowl, stir together the barbecue sauce, smoked paprika, and salt; set aside.
2. In a large saucepan over medium heat, fully heat the oil. Add the popcorn kernels, cover with a lid, and periodically shake the saucepan until you hear the popping begin. Let the popcorn pop undisturbed until it stops, about 3 minutes. Carefully remove lid.
3. Immediately drizzle the barbecue sauce mixture onto popcorn while over medium heat. Stir well (or shake) until the popcorn is lightly coated and re-crisped, about 2 minutes.
4. Sprinkle with the nutritional yeast and serve while warm.

NUTRITION INFO

Choices/Exchanges: 1½ starch, 1 fat

Per serving: 160 calories, 7 g total fat, 1 g saturated fat, 0 g trans fat, 0 mg cholesterol, 220 mg sodium, 111 mg potassium, 19 g total carbohydrate, 4 g dietary fiber, 1 g sugars, 0 g added sugars, 4 g protein, 50 mg phosphorus

Popcorn Is "See" Food

Though they might get stuck in between your teeth, you'll definitely want to appreciate those little popcorn hulls. They're loaded with plant nutrients, including lutein and zeaxanthin. These carotenoids may play a key role in keeping your eyes healthy.

FRUIT-SWEETENED BBQ SAUCE

- ¼ cup fruit-sweetened or no-sugar-added ketchup
- 3 tablespoons unsweetened applesauce
- 1 teaspoon apple cider vinegar
- ½ teaspoon freshly ground black pepper
- ½ teaspoon smoked paprika

In a liquid measuring cup, stir together all ingredients. Serve, or store in a sealed jar in the refrigerator for up to 1 week. Makes 4 servings, about 2 tablespoons each.

NUTRITION INFO
Choices/Exchanges = 0
Per serving: 15 calories, 0 g total fat, 0 g saturated fat, 0 g trans fat, 0 mg cholesterol, 105 mg sodium, 60 mg potassium, 4 g total carbohydrate, 0 g dietary fiber, 0 g sugars, 0 g added sugars, 0 g protein, 5 mg phosphorus

PARTY HUMMUS CANAPÉS

If you're looking for a festive party pleaser, these fun canapés will delight your guests—even the picky ones. They look impressive, yet they're so easy to fix. For a soirée, try this: Measure 1 cup of hummus and count out 16 pita chips and roasted chickpea snacks in advance, then arrange in just a couple of minutes at party time. If you choose to make these finger food apps really quickly using packaged hummus, go organic—or read the ingredient list and select one without synthetic preservatives, such as potassium sorbate. These preservatives can make some hummus brands last longer, but your body simply doesn't need them!

SERVES: 8 | SERVING SIZE: 2 canapés
PREP TIME: 8 minutes | COOK TIME: 0 minutes

- 16 whole-grain or multigrain pita chips
- 1 cup hummus of choice (see recipes in this book)
- 16 fresh cilantro leaves
- 16 crunchy roasted chickpea snacks (plain or flavored) or *Wild Buffalo Chickpea Snackers* (page 55)
- Pinch of smoked paprika or roasted sesame seeds

DIRECTIONS

1. Top each pita chip with 1 tablespoon hummus and place onto a platter.
2. Place a cilantro leaf and roasted chickpea on top of each.
3. Dust (lightly sprinkle) with smoked paprika or sesame seeds and serve.

NUTRITION INFO

Choices/Exchanges: ½ starch, 1 fat

Per serving: 80 calories, 4 g total fat, 0.6 g saturated fat, 0 g trans fat, 0 mg cholesterol, 170 mg sodium, 85 mg potassium, 9 g total carbohydrate, 3 g dietary fiber, 2 g sugars, 0 g added sugars, 3 g protein, 65 mg phosphorus

Appetizing Variations

Need kid-friendlier finger foods? Top these with thinly sliced grape tomatoes instead of the cilantro and chickpeas. Prefer to go lower carb (or your party guests are all veggie radicals!)? Enjoy the hummus on sliced, fresh English cucumber "chips" instead of pita chips and top with extra thinly sliced, red hot chili peppers instead of chickpeas.

JACKIE'S CLASSIC HUMMUS

- 1 (15-ounce) can no-salt-added chickpeas (garbanzo beans), drained
- 1/3 cup tahini
- 3 to 4 tablespoons unsweetened green tea, chilled
- Juice of 1 small lemon (2 tablespoons)
- 1 large garlic clove, chopped
- ¾ teaspoon sea salt, or to taste
- ¼ teaspoon ground cumin
- 1/8 teaspoon ground cayenne pepper (optional)

DIRECTIONS

Add all of the ingredients to a food processor or blender. Cover, purée until velvety smooth (at least 2 minutes), and serve. (Makes 7 servings, ¼ cup each, when eaten as a dip.)

NUTRITION INFO

Choices/Exchanges: 1 Starch, 1 Fat

Per serving: 130 calories, 7 g total fat, 1 g saturated fat, 0 g trans fat, 0 mg cholesterol, 260 mg sodium, 190 mg potassium, 12 g total carbohydrate, 3 g dietary fiber, 0 g sugars, 0 g added sugars, 5 g protein, 142 mg phosphorus

PULSE PARTY NACHOS

When you're having friends or family over for a football watch party or other casual gathering, you'll definitely want this popular, party-worthy recipe on the menu. It tastes absolutely meaty thanks to the zesty topping made with the trio of sautéed black beans, walnuts, and baby bellas. Using pulse-based tortilla chips powers up the protein and intrigue. And all of the add-ons, including crisp lettuce, plant-based sour cream, red hot chili pepper, and fresh cilantro, make it extra flavorful. It's a real showstopper—and so much fun to share.

SERVES: 10 I SERVING SIZE: 1 cup
PREP TIME: 25 minutes I COOK TIME: 15 minutes

- 2 teaspoons avocado oil or sunflower oil
- 12 ounces baby bellas (crimini mushrooms), finely chopped
- 1/3 cup finely chopped walnuts (1.5 ounces)
- 1/3 cup diced red onion
- 1 (14.5-ounce) can fire-roasted diced tomatoes (do not drain)
- 1 (15-ounce) can no-salt-added black beans or lentils, drained
- 1 lime cut into 6 wedges, divided
- ¾ teaspoon ground cumin
- ¾ teaspoon chili powder
- ¼ teaspoon + 1/8 teaspoon sea salt
- 1 cup shredded, plant-based Mexican-style cheese* (4 ounces)
- 8 ounces chickpea, black bean, or whole-grain corn tortilla chips, divided
- ½ cup packed shredded romaine lettuce
- 1/3 cup plant-based sour cream or *Avocado Crema* (page 33)
- ¼ cup loosely packed fresh cilantro leaves
- 1 small red hot chili pepper, extra thinly sliced

**Note: Ideally, choose vegan cheese products based on tree nuts.*

DIRECTIONS

1. Heat the oil in a large cast-iron skillet or wok over medium-high heat. Add the mushrooms, walnuts, and onion and sauté until the mushrooms are fully wilted, about 7 minutes.

2. Add the tomatoes, beans, juice of 3 lime wedges (1 tablespoon juice), cumin, chili powder, and salt and sauté until no excess liquid remains, about 7 minutes. Sprinkle with the plant-based cheese.
3. Add half of the tortilla chips to a platter, top with half of the bean mixture, then add the remaining tortillas and bean mixture. Top with the lettuce, sour cream, cilantro, and chili pepper. Serve immediately with the remaining lime wedges.

NUTRITION INFO

Choices/Exchanges: 2 carbohydrate, 1 lean protein, 2 fat

Per serving: 240 calories, 12 g total fat, 1.5 g saturated fat, 0 g trans fat, 0 mg cholesterol, 360 mg sodium, 464 mg potassium, 27 g total carbohydrate, 8 g dietary fiber, 2 g sugars, 0 g added sugars, 8 g protein, 94 mg phosphorus

Why Use a Cast-Iron Skillet?

If your cooktop works with a cast-iron pan, it's an ideal choice for preparing foods without adding excess oils (aka excess calories), since the surface is stick-resistant and improves over time. Plus, eating food prepared in a cast-iron skillet naturally increases the amount of iron you'll be getting.

Pulse-Based Tortilla Chips

Generally speaking, pulses are dry beans, peas, chickpeas, and lentils. Instead of being made with ground corn, tortilla chips can be based on these pulses. So if you want to power up your protein intake, try black bean or chickpea tortilla chips with this recipe—and beyond.

Main Dishes: Breakfasts and Brunches

SAVORY HERBED MEDITERRANEAN OATMEAL

While oatmeal is often served in a sweet way, your taste buds will be thrilled to meet its savory side. Treat yourself to this clever morning main dish designed just for one. Think of it like a creamy risotto, but oats instead of arborio rice is the grain of choice. The sun-dried tomatoes provide an eye-opening pop of umami (that "meaty" sense of taste). And plant-based goat cheese and basil provide a lovely finishing touch. After discovering (or re-discovering) this savory way to prepare oatmeal, you might not want to go back to a sweetened bowl of it again.

SERVES: 1 I SERVING SIZE: 1 rounded cup
PREP TIME: 12 minutes I COOK TIME: 5 minutes

- 1 cup low-sodium vegetable broth
- 4 large sun-dried tomato halves, not oil-packed, thinly sliced (do not rehydrate)
- ⅛ teaspoon sea salt, or to taste
- ⅛ teaspoon freshly ground black pepper
- ½ cup old-fashioned, whole-grain, rolled oats
- 1½ tablespoons minced fresh chives
- 3 tablespoons plain, unsweetened, plant-based, Greek-style yogurt

- 1½ tablespoons crumbled, plain, plant-based, goat-style cheese or other vegan cheese*
- 1 tablespoon thinly sliced fresh basil or 6 small fresh basil leaves

**Note: Ideally, choose vegan cheese products based on tree nuts.*

DIRECTIONS

1. Bring the broth, sun-dried tomatoes, salt and pepper to a boil in a small saucepan.
2. Stir in the oats and chives and reduce heat to medium. Stir until the oats are fully cooked, about 5 minutes. Remove from the heat and stir in the plant-based yogurt. Adjust seasoning.
3. Transfer to a bowl, sprinkle with the plant-based cheese and basil, and serve.

NUTRITION INFO

Choices/Exchanges: 2 starch, 1 lean protein, 2 fat

Per serving: 290 calories, 9 g total fat, 1.5 g saturated fat, 0 g trans fat, 0 mg cholesterol, 530 mg sodium, 573 mg potassium, 39 g total carbohydrate, 6 g dietary fiber, 6 g sugars, 0 g added sugars, 13 g protein, 263 mg phosphorus

What Is Plant-Based, Greek-Style Yogurt?

While yogurt is classically a dairy food, there are now many non-dairy options to choose from. Instead of cow's milk, they're based on plant milk, such as almond milk. For thickening, you might find the addition of a starch, like tapioca starch. For the equivalent protein, soy protein isolate might be included. However, the key thing to look for on the ingredient label is "live active cultures"—these are the good-for-your-gut bacteria that make the product act like yogurt.

BREAKFAST VEGGIE TACOS

Turn tofu likers into lovers with these tacos. Here, tofu acts and looks so much like scrambled eggs, making it an ideal filling for tortillas. All of the aromatic herbs and spices create flavor appeal. For bonus interest, try with a combo of zucchini and yellow squash; spread with the velvety *Avocado Crema;* or consider using a flavored tofu, like extra-firm spinach-jalapeño tofu. Whichever way you stuff these soft tacos (you get two for a serving!), they create a fully satisfying meal on their own. The trio of protein, fiber, and veggie volume will carry you through to lunch. In fact, enjoy these tacos at lunchtime, too!

SERVES: 4 | SERVING SIZE: 2 tacos
PREP TIME: 25 minutes (doesn't include guacamole prep time) | COOK TIME: 13 minutes

- ¾ cup *Jackie's Hass Avocado Guacamole* (page 90) or *Avocado Crema* (page 33)
- 8 (6-inch) soft, whole-grain corn tortillas
- 1 tablespoon avocado oil or unrefined peanut oil
- 3 scallions, green and white parts, thinly sliced
- 2 medium (7 ounces each) zucchini or yellow squash, finely diced (2½ cups)
- 1 large (4.5-ounce) poblano pepper, minced
- 1 (14-ounce) package extra-firm organic tofu,* drained and gently squeezed of excess liquid, finely diced
- 1 teaspoon ground cumin
- ½ teaspoon finely chopped fresh oregano leaves
- ½ teaspoon sea salt, or to taste
- ¼ teaspoon ground turmeric
- 1 cup cherry tomatoes, quartered
- Juice of ½ lime (1 tablespoon)
- 3 tablespoons chopped fresh cilantro and 8 fresh cilantro sprigs

**Note: Use tofu that's made from soybeans (traditional), chickpeas, or pumpkin seeds.*

DIRECTIONS

1. Spread 1½ tablespoons of the guacamole onto each tortilla. Set aside.
2. Heat the oil in a large skillet over medium-high heat. Add the scallions, zucchini, and poblano pepper and sauté for 2 minutes.
3. Add the tofu, cumin, oregano, salt, and turmeric and sauté until the zucchini is tender, about 8 minutes. Stir in the tomatoes and lime juice and sauté until the tomatoes are heated through, about 2 minutes. Stir in the chopped cilantro. Adjust seasoning.
4. Spoon the tofu-veggie mixture down the center of each tortilla, about ½ cup each. Top each with a cilantro sprig, fold, and serve.

NUTRITION INFO

Choices/Exchanges: 1½ starch, 2 vegetable, 1 lean protein, 2 fat

Per serving: 310 calories, 16 g total fat, 2 g saturated fat, 0 g trans fat, 0 mg cholesterol, 410 mg sodium, 530 mg potassium, 31 g total carbohydrate, 9 g dietary fiber, 5 g sugars, 0 g added sugars, 15 g protein, 180 mg phosphorus

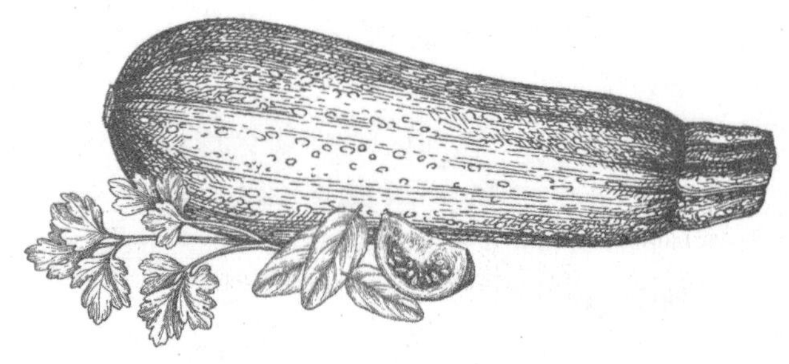

ROASTED CAULIFLOWER STEAK FLORENTINE

A beauty of a breakfast or brunch! This nutritious, plant-based interpretation of eggs Florentine features impressive, steak-like slabs of caramelized cauliflower in place of English muffin, oozy roasted tomato instead of poached egg, and a scrumptious, velvety, vegan sauce instead of über rich hollandaise. The pinch of sumac provides lip-smacking tang, though the touch of heat from cayenne works equally well. The bonus: by increasing your veggie intake, you may have a better chance at managing or decreasing your weight.

SERVES: 4 | SERVING SIZE: 1 topped cauliflower steak
PREP TIME: 30 minutes (includes sauce prep time) | COOK TIME: 50 minutes (includes sauce cook time)

- 4 (1-inch thick) whole slices from a large head cauliflower* (about 6 ½ ounces per slice)
- 2 medium vine-ripened tomatoes, halved crosswise
- 1 tablespoon extra-virgin olive oil
- ¼ teaspoon sea salt, divided
- 5 cups packed fresh baby spinach (5 ounces)
- 5 cups packed fresh leafy greens of choice, such as tatsoi (5 ounces)
- Juice of ½ small lemon (1 tablespoon)
- ⅛ teaspoon freshly grated or ground nutmeg
- ¾ cup *Hollandaise-Style Sauce,* warm (see recipe that follows)
- ⅛ teaspoon ground sumac or cayenne pepper, or to taste

DIRECTIONS

1. Preheat the oven to 450°F. Brush the cauliflower slices and tomato halves with the oil and arrange on a large baking sheet lined with a silicone baking mat or unbleached parchment paper.
2. Roast until the cauliflower and tomato halves are lightly caramelized, about 20 minutes. Gently flip over just the cauliflower. Sprinkle the cauliflower and tomato halves with ⅛ teaspoon of the salt. Roast until the cauliflower is fully caramelized and tomatoes are fully roasted, about 18 minutes more.
3. Meanwhile, add the spinach and leafy greens to a stockpot or large deep skillet over medium heat. Cover and steam until all greens are fully wilted, about 8 minutes, stirring twice. (Note: The greens will wilt down to about 1⅓ cups.) Add the lemon juice,

nutmeg, and the remaining ⅛ teaspoon salt. Transfer the greens to a fine mesh strainer to gently drain excess liquids.

4. Top each cauliflower slice with about ⅓ cup of the greens, a roasted tomato half, and 3 tablespoons of the sauce. Sprinkle with the sumac. Serve immediately.

**With a chef's knife, slice down from the top of the cauliflower head through the stem end. If you're unable to find a large head of cauliflower (2 pounds or larger), use 2 medium heads and cut slices slightly thicker (about 2 slices per cauliflower head). Use the largest center slices for this dish. Reserve the remaining cauliflower for other use, such as in* Chimichurri Hummus and Cauliflower Wrap (page 145) *or* Vegetable Mousse "Meatloaf." (page 117)

NUTRITION INFO
Choices/Exchanges: 1 carbohydrate, 2 vegetable, 1 fat
Per serving: 160 calories, 7 g total fat, 1 g saturated fat, 0 g trans fat, 0 mg cholesterol, 490 mg sodium, 460 mg potassium, 20 g total carbohydrate, 9 g dietary fiber, 6 g sugars, 0 g added sugars, 8 g protein, 90 mg phosphorus

HOLLANDAISE-STYLE SAUCE

- ½ cup silken organic tofu, drained
- 2 tablespoons plain, unsweetened plant-based milk of choice
- Juice and zest of 1 small lemon (2 tablespoons juice)
- 1 tablespoon creamy, raw, no-salt-added almond butter or tahini
- 1½ teaspoons spicy brown mustard
- ¾ teaspoon vegetarian Worcestershire sauce, or to taste
- ¼ teaspoon hot Madras curry powder, or to taste
- ¼ teaspoon sea salt, or to taste

DIRECTIONS

1. Add the tofu, plant-based milk, lemon juice, almond butter, mustard, Worcestershire sauce, curry powder, and salt to a blender. Cover and purée until smooth.
2. Pour the tofu mixture into a small saucepan over medium heat. Simmer while stirring until fully heated, about 3 minutes. Stir in desired amount of the lemon zest and adjust seasoning. If preferred, reserve some zest for garnishing. Serve while warm in *Roasted Cauliflower Steak Florentine.* (Makes ¾ cup sauce; 4 servings, 3 tablespoons each.)

NUTRITION INFO
Choices/Exchanges: ½ fat
Per serving: 45 calories, 3 g total fat, 0 g saturated fat, 0 g trans fat, 0 mg cholesterol, 210 mg sodium, 46 mg potassium, 2 g total carbohydrate, 1 g dietary fiber, 1 g sugars, 0 g added sugars, 2 g protein, 22 mg phosphorus

CHILAQUILES-STYLE BOWL

Chilaquiles are a classic Mexican dish that features tortilla chips simmered in salsa. This version goes heavy on the add-ins—including pinto beans and vegan eggs—and is fully plant-based. If you can't find a plant-based egg alternative, use mashed chickpeas or *Squashed Chickpea "Eggs" with Plant-Based Goat Cheese* (page 71) in its place. Either way, think of this flavorful, fun, and filling recipe like scrambled-up breakfast tacos. *Delicioso!*

SERVES: 4 I SERVING SIZE: 1 rounded cup
PREP TIME: 15 minutes I COOK TIME: 6 minutes

- 1 cup liquid plant-based eggs
- ¼ cup + 2 tablespoons medium or mild tomatillo salsa (salsa verde)
- ¾ teaspoon finely chopped fresh oregano leaves
- 1½ teaspoons avocado oil or peanut oil
- 1 cup cooked or drained canned pinto or black beans, patted dry
- 16 whole-grain corn tortilla chips or pulse-based tortilla chips, whole or broken
- 1 small Hass avocado, peeled, pitted and diced
- Pinch of sea salt
- 2 tablespoons plant-based sour cream
- ¼ cup loosely packed fresh cilantro leaves

DIRECTIONS

1. In a medium bowl, stir together the plant-based eggs, 2 tablespoons of the tomatillo salsa, and the oregano.
2. Heat the oil in a large, stick-resistant skillet over medium heat. Add the plant-based egg mixture and cook while gently stirring until softly scrambled, about 4 minutes. Fold in the beans and chips until the beans are heated through, about 1 minute.
3. Transfer the chilaquiles-style mixture to individual bowls. Sprinkle with the avocado, salt, plant-based sour cream, and cilantro leaves. Serve with the remaining ¼ cup tomatillo salsa on the side.

NUTRITION INFO

Choices/Exchanges: 1½ starch, 1 lean protein, 2½ fat

Per serving: 280 calories, 16 g total fat, 1.5 g saturated fat, 0 g trans fat, 0 mg cholesterol, 460 mg sodium, 398 mg potassium, 23 g total carbohydrate, 6 g dietary fiber, 1 g sugars, 0 g added sugars, 12 g protein, 108 mg phosphorus

Almost Cowboy Caviar

When you open a can of beans, like black, pinto, or kidney beans, and don't need to use the entire amount right way, make this with the extras. Just stir together ½ cup each drained beans, thawed frozen sweet corn (or prepared corn), fresh pico de gallo, and, if you like, diced avocado. Serve it as a zippy salad or salsa.

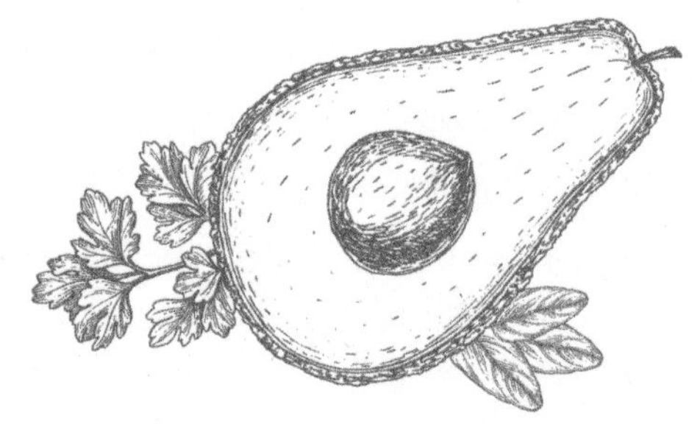

SQUASHED CHICKPEA "EGGS" WITH PLANT-BASED GOAT CHEESE

It can seem challenging to get a good source of protein for breakfast or brunch when following a diabetes-friendly, 100-percent plant-based eating plan. But if you're a fan of chickpeas, you're in luck. Here they're served just like scrambled eggs—only tastier! The array of spices creates cuisine drama. The yellow summer squash offers more volume while helping you get your veggies. And the finishing touch of plant-based goat cheese offers tangy, creamy comfort. This recipe is extra inviting paired with plant-based bacon.

SERVES: 3 | SERVING SIZE: ¾ cup
PREP TIME: 15 minutes | COOK TIME: 10 minutes

- 1 (15-ounce) can no-salt-added chickpeas (garbanzo beans)
- 2 tablespoons nutritional yeast flakes
- ½ teaspoon + ⅛ teaspoon ground turmeric
- ½ teaspoon sea salt, or to taste
- ¼ teaspoon smoked paprika
- ¼ teaspoon garlic powder
- ¼ teaspoon freshly ground black pepper
- 1 tablespoon extra-virgin olive oil
- 1 medium (8-ounce) yellow summer squash, small diced
- 1 ounce (2 tablespoons) plain, plant-based, goat-style cheese or other soft vegan cheese*
- 2 tablespoons chopped fresh chives or small fresh basil leaves, or to taste

**Note: Ideally, choose vegan cheese products based on tree nuts.*

DIRECTIONS

1. Drain the chickpeas, reserving ¼ cup of the liquid from the can.
2. To a medium bowl, add the drained chickpeas and ¼ cup chickpea liquid. Smash with a large fork until the mixture is slightly lumpy and resembles scrambled eggs. Stir in the nutritional yeast, turmeric, salt, paprika, garlic powder, and pepper until evenly combined. Set aside.

3. Heat the olive oil in a large cast-iron or other stick-resistant skillet over medium-high heat. Add the squash and sauté until it's lightly browned, about 5 minutes. Add the smashed chickpea mixture and sauté/scramble until the mixture is lightly browned, about 4 minutes.
4. Transfer the "eggs" to a platter. Top with little dollops of the plant-based, goat-style cheese, sprinkle with the chives, and serve.

NUTRITION INFO

Choices/Exchanges: 1 starch, 2 vegetable, 1 high fat protein

Per serving: 250 calories, 8 g total fat, 1 g saturated fat, 0 g trans fat, 0 mg cholesterol, 460 mg sodium, 570 mg potassium, 30 g total carbohydrate, 8 g dietary fiber, 3 g sugars, 0 g added sugars, 13 g protein, 174 mg phosphorus

Time-Saving Tip

Need a quicker fix first thing in the morning? Follow steps 1 and 2 in the evening and stash the mixture in the fridge. Then when you wake up in the morning, remove from the fridge and start with step 3. Need it even speedier? Simply make this entire recipe in the evening and reheat in a skillet or microwave in the morning. It tastes just as good.

Chickpea Aquafaba

The slightly thickened liquid that remains from cooked or canned beans is called aquafaba. Chickpea aquafaba has just a hint of the bean flavor, making it versatile in recipes. While there are thousands of uses for it, one of my favorites is to transform it into an aquafaba "mayo" (it looks and tastes like classic mayo!). Using an electric blender, I make it by blending together ¼ cup aquafaba, ⅔ cup sunflower oil, 1½ teaspoons lemon juice, 1 teaspoon each white balsamic vinegar and yellow mustard, and sea salt to taste.

AVOCADO AND GARBANZO SMASH TOASTS

Are you an avocado toast fan? You'll love this duo of smashed avocado and garbanzo bean toasts. The toppings aren't just spread like butter onto the toasted whole-grain bread; ideally, they're piled high into luxurious mounds. The garnish of pistachios, smoked paprika, and fresh chives make them wow-worthy. And as a bonus, you'll get a punch of plant protein to make this a meal worth repeating regularly.

SERVES: 1 | SERVING SIZE: 2 topped toast halves
PREP TIME: 12 minutes | COOK TIME: 2 minutes (for toasting bread)

- ⅓ cup canned, drained, no-salt-added chickpeas (garbanzo beans)
- 2 teaspoons extra-virgin olive oil
- 2 teaspoons lemon juice, divided
- ⅛ teaspoon sea salt, divided
- ⅓ cup mashed Hass avocado (from about ½ avocado)
- 1 large slice whole-grain bread, toasted and halved
- 1 tablespoon shelled, lightly salted, roasted pistachios
- ⅛ teaspoon ground smoked paprika
- 2 teaspoons minced fresh chives

DIRECTIONS

1. In a small bowl, using a fork or potato masher, gently smash the chickpeas with the olive oil, 1 teaspoon of the lemon juice, and a pinch of the salt.
2. In a separate small bowl, stir together the mashed avocado, the remaining 1 teaspoon lemon juice, and remaining pinch of salt.
3. Top one toast half with the chickpea mixture. Top the other toast half with the avocado mixture. Sprinkle both toasts with the pistachios, paprika, and chives. Enjoy with a fork and knife.

NUTRITION INFO

Choices/Exchanges: 3 starch, 1 high fat protein, 2½ fat

Per serving: 450 calories, 26 g total fat, 3.5 g saturated fat, 0 g trans fat, 0 mg cholesterol, 490 mg sodium, 721 mg potassium, 42 g total carbohydrate, 9 g dietary fiber, 5 g sugars, 0 g added sugars, 13 g protein, 239 mg phosphorus

Extra Avocado? Extra Chickpeas?

You can always plan to toss any extra avocado or chickpeas onto a salad—or reserve them to make these toasts again tomorrow. Here are a few other scrumptious ideas. Mash up those spare chickpeas with a little salsa or salsa verde and enjoy in recipes as "cheater" refried beans. Dice up any remaining avocado and stir in a little salsa verde or pico de gallo to enjoy as "lazy" guacamole. Or make something with both avocado and chickpea extras, like avocado hummus that uses avocado in place of some of the chickpeas in a classic hummus recipe. It's so good!

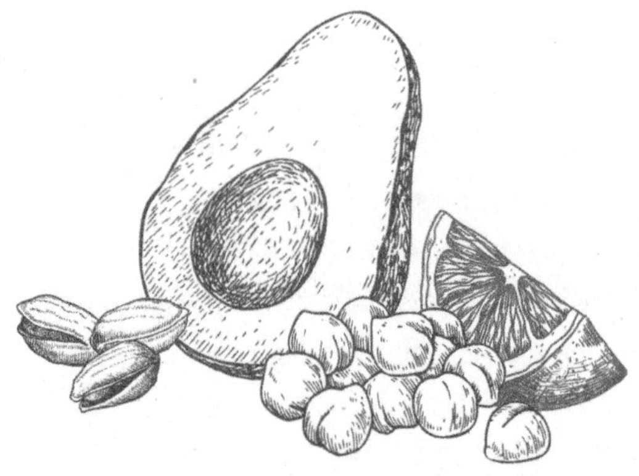

BELL PEPPER, SWEET POTATO AND "SAUSAGE" HASH SKILLET

A carb-friendlier way to do hash browns is to give bell peppers the starring role. A more colorful and antioxidant-packed way to do them is to use sweet potato instead of potato, choose at least two different colored peppers, and finish with fresh herbs. And to make them extra scrumptious, add sausage—or, in this instance, plant-based sausage. If you like, make this skillet with chorizo-style seitan instead of plant-based sausage for a change of taste. It's a breakfast side dish full of taste bud wow.

SERVES: 4 | SERVING SIZE: about 1 cup
PREP TIME: 15 minutes | COOK TIME: 27 minutes

- 1 (3.5-ounce) link uncooked plant-based Italian-style sausage (or chorizo-style seitan)
- 1½ tablespoons extra-virgin olive oil, divided
- 1 large (10- to 11-ounce) unpeeled sweet potato, scrubbed, ends trimmed, cut into ½-inch cubes
- 1 large green bell pepper, cubed
- 1 large red bell pepper, cubed
- 1 small hot chili pepper, with some seeds, extra thinly sliced
- ¼ teaspoon + ⅛ teaspoon sea salt, or to taste
- ⅛ teaspoon smoked paprika
- 1½ teaspoons red wine vinegar
- ¼ cup packed, thinly sliced, fresh chives or scallions
- ¼ cup packed, roughly chopped, fresh flat-leaf parsley

DIRECTIONS

1. Prepare the plant-based sausage according to package directions. When cool enough to handle, thinly slice into coins. Set aside.
2. Meanwhile, in a large (12-inch) cast iron or other stick-resistant skillet, fully heat 1 tablespoon of the olive oil over medium heat. Stir in the sweet potato, cover, and cook until slightly softened and lightly browned, about 7 minutes, stirring twice.
3. Add the bell peppers, hot pepper, salt, paprika, and the remaining ½ tablespoon olive oil, increase heat to medium-high, and cook uncovered while stirring occasionally

until the vegetables are browned as desired, about 8 minutes. Stir in the sausage and vinegar until heated through, about 1 minute.

4. Remove from heat, stir in the chives and parsley, adjust seasoning, and serve.

NUTRITION INFO

Choices/Exchanges: 1 starch, 1 vegetable, 1½ fat

Per serving: 170 calories, 9 g total fat, 2.5 g saturated fat, 0 g trans fat, 0 mg cholesterol, 410 mg sodium, 498 mg potassium, 17 g total carbohydrate, 4 g dietary fiber, 6 g sugars, 0 g added sugars, 7 g protein, 51 mg phosphorus

From Side Dish to Main Dish

This hash skillet is designed to be served as a side. But if you'd like to do a one-skillet meal, simply push the hash to the sides of the skillet after stirring in the plant-based sausage in step 3. Scramble vegan eggs in the center of the skillet. Then stir everything together. Alternatively, stir in a can of rinsed, drained, reduced-sodium black beans along with the plant-based sausage in step 3.

PLANT-BASED BREAKFAST SAUSAGE PATTIES

The taste, aroma, and appearance of these patties are all reminiscent of breakfast sausage. But this plant-based version of breakfast sausage patties is based on eggplant and baby bellas to give you veggie goodness with plenty of heartiness—and without greasiness. The recipe is easier than it looks, too. Many of the ingredients in this recipe are spices which take little time to measure. Want to make it in advance? Chill the prepared patties in the fridge overnight, then simply reheat in the microwave, skillet, or oven at breakfast- or brunch-time.

SERVES: 4 | SERVING SIZE: 3 patties
PREP TIME: 22 minutes | COOK TIME: 33 to 35 minutes

- 1 tablespoon chia seeds
- 3 tablespoons no-sugar-added marinara sauce
- ½ cup old-fashioned, whole-grain rolled oats
- 1 tablespoon + 2 teaspoons extra-virgin olive oil, divided
- 1 small (12-ounce) eggplant with peel, stem removed, small diced (4 cups diced)
- 4 ounces baby bellas (crimini mushrooms), finely chopped
- 2 garlic cloves, minced
- 1 teaspoon minced fresh thyme leaves
- 1 teaspoon minced fresh rosemary leaves
- ¾ teaspoon ground sage
- ½ teaspoon sea salt, or to taste
- ½ teaspoon fennel seeds
- ¼ teaspoon freshly ground black pepper
- ⅛ teaspoon ground nutmeg
- Pinch of ground cayenne pepper
- 1½ tablespoons nutritional yeast flakes

DIRECTIONS

1. In a small bowl, stir together the chia seeds and marinara sauce. Set aside.
2. Add the oats to a food processor and pulse several times to finely chop (do not process into flour). Set aside.
3. Preheat the oven to 400°F. Line a large rimmed baking sheet with a silicone baking mat or unbleached parchment paper.

4. Heat 1 tablespoon of the olive oil in a large, deep, cast-iron skillet or a wok over medium-high heat. Add the eggplant, baby bellas, garlic, thyme, rosemary, sage, salt, fennel seeds, black pepper, nutmeg, and cayenne and cook while stirring occasionally until the veggies are browned and fully softened, about 11 minutes. Transfer the mixture to a medium mixing bowl.
5. Add the chia marinara to the eggplant-baby bella mixture; stir to combine. Add the chopped oats and nutritional yeast; stir to combine. Set aside to slightly cool for 5 minutes.
6. Form the mixture into 12 round mounds, about 2 tablespoons each, on the prepared baking sheet. (Hint: Use a medium cookie scoop.) Press into 2-inch diameter patties. Lightly brush the tops of the patties with the remaining 2 teaspoons olive oil, and roast until browned, about 20 to 22 minutes.
7. Remove from the oven and set aside to complete the cooking process and firm up, about 5 minutes. Enjoy with a fork.

NUTRITION INFO
Choices/Exchanges: 1 starch, 1 vegetable, 1 fat
Per serving: 150 calories, 8 g total fat, 1 g saturated fat, 0 g trans fat, 0 mg cholesterol, 340 mg sodium, 489 mg potassium, 18 g total carbohydrate, 5 g dietary fiber, 4 g sugars, 0 g added sugars, 5 g protein, 112 mg phosphorus

Super Seeds

White and black chia seeds are super nutritious—and super cool. They create a gel when in liquid for about 10 minutes. So, when making recipes that use chia seeds in this way, make sure you plan time into your prep to allow the seeds to gel. Choose white chia seeds for a prettier appearance in light-colored recipes. In this recipe, any color works. Bonus: chia seeds are a great source of fiber and protein. This can help prevent sharp spikes in blood glucose since it can help whatever they're paired with convert into sugar more slowly in the body.

Breakfast Sausage Spice Mixture

For a quicker fix, make breakfast sausage seasoning in advance. Combine ¾ teaspoon ground sage, ½ teaspoon sea salt, ½ teaspoon fennel seeds, ¼ teaspoon freshly ground black pepper, ⅛ teaspoon ground nutmeg, and a pinch of ground cayenne pepper in a jar, seal, label, and stash in the pantry. Double or triple these ingredients if you plan to make this recipe regularly. Then use 2⅛ teaspoons of this spice mixture when preparing the recipe.

SMOKY PORTABELLA BACON

These plant-based portabella bacon strips are a must try for a special occasion! They're basically thinly sliced portabella mushroom caps, brushed with olive oil, and sprinkled with spices, sea salt, and a just-right amount of natural sugar for taste balance, and then baked low and slow until crisp. These strips are delightfully salty—so be sure to not go overboard on sodium the rest of the day. Enjoy just like regular bacon—and in *Portabella BLT Sandwich with Heirloom Tomatoes* (page 151) or paired with *Squashed Chickpea "Eggs" with Plant-Based Goat Cheese* (page 71).

SERVES: 4 | SERVING SIZE: 12 strips
PREP TIME: 8 minutes | COOK TIME: 2 hours 15 minutes

- 2 large (5- to 6-inch diameter) portabella mushroom caps, extra-thinly sliced (about 48 total slices)
- 2 tablespoons extra-virgin olive oil
- 1½ tablespoons coconut sugar
- ¾ teaspoon smoked paprika
- ¾ teaspoon sea salt
- ¾ teaspoon freshly ground black pepper, or to taste
- ½ teaspoon chipotle or classic chili powder

DIRECTIONS

1. Preheat the oven to 275°F. Line two baking sheets with silicone baking mats or unbleached parchment paper.
2. Arrange the portabella strips on the baking sheets in a single layer. Lightly brush just the top side of each strip with the olive oil.
3. In a small bowl, stir together the sugar, paprika, salt, pepper, and chili powder. (Hint: For a milder version, use less black pepper.) Generously and evenly sprinkle all of the spice mixture over each portabella strip.
4. Roast for 1 hour 30 minutes, then turn off the oven and let the portabella bacon crisp in the oven for 45 minutes. Cool on the baking sheets on a cooling rack to further crisp.

NUTRITION INFO
Choices/Exchanges: 1 vegetable, 1½ fat
Per serving: 90 calories, 7 g total fat, 1 g saturated fat, 0 g trans fat, 0 mg cholesterol, 460 mg sodium, 196 mg potassium, 7 g total carbohydrate, 1 g dietary fiber, 6 g sugars, 0 g added sugars, 1 g protein, 48 mg phosphorus

Make-Ahead Tip

If you want to enjoy this crisped plant-based bacon early in the morning, consider preparing it in advance due to the baking time required. If you do, place the fully baked and cooled strips in a sealable container in the refrigerator overnight. In the morning, simply set the strips out for 20 minutes to bring to room temperature. Or reheat in a dry skillet over medium heat for 1½ to 2 minutes per side, then let cool for a few minutes to allow to re-crisp.

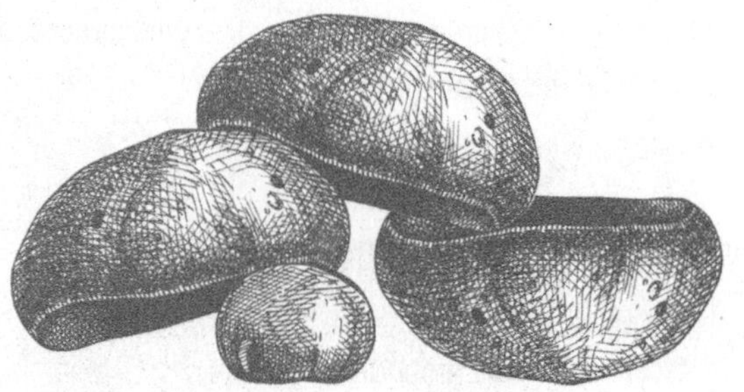

COCOA-COVERED STRAWBERRY OVERNIGHT OATMEAL

This fiber-packed overnight oatmeal offers "sweet treat" appeal but in a good-for-you way. The plant-based, Greek-style yogurt makes it extra creamy. The combination of strawberry fruit spread and sliced strawberries makes the fruitiness pop. And the finishing cocoa powder provides "chocolate-covered strawberry" vibes. Prepare it in the evening (or even a couple days in advance), then in the morning . . . just grab a spoon and dig in!

SERVES: 1 | SERVING SIZE: 1 jar
PREP TIME: 8 minutes (plus overnight chilling) | COOK TIME: 8 minutes

- ⅓ cup old-fashioned, whole-grain rolled oats
- ⅓ cup vanilla, unsweetened, plant-based milk
- ⅓ cup plain, unsweetened, plant-based Greek-style yogurt
- 1 tablespoon fruit-sweetened strawberry fruit spread (jam)*
- 7 fresh or thawed frozen strawberries, stems removed and thinly sliced
- 1 teaspoon unsweetened cocoa powder

**Note: Ideally, choose a fruit spread without added sugars.*

DIRECTIONS

1. Add the oats, plant-based milk, and plant-based yogurt to a 1½-cup-capacity jar or sealable container. Stir well.
2. Top the oat mixture with the fruit spread, sliced strawberries, and cocoa.
3. Seal the jar with a lid. Chill in the refrigerator overnight, at least 6 hours. Serve.

NUTRITION INFO

Choices/Exchanges: 1 starch, 1½ fruit, 1 medium fat protein

Per serving: 240 calories, 6 g total fat, 1 g saturated fat, 0 g trans fat, 0 mg cholesterol, 140 mg sodium, 402 mg potassium, 37 g total carbohydrate, 6 g dietary fiber, 12 g sugars, 0 g added sugars, 12 g protein, 140 mg phosphorus

Grab-N-Go

Make a few jars in advance for an on-the-go breakfast throughout the week. This oatmeal can be stored in the fridge for up to 4 days.

Plant-Based Milk Alternatives

There are so many plant-based milk options, including flax, oat, almond, brown rice, and peanut milk. Choose an unsweetened one for this recipe. If you can't find an unsweetened variety that's vanilla flavored, add ¼ teaspoon pure vanilla extract to ⅓ cup plain, unsweetened, plant-based milk of choice for use in this recipe.

HOMEMADE GRANOLA-RASPBERRY JARS

Hey vegetarians (and nonvegetarians), this parfait-in-a-jar is for you. In other words, it's for everyone! It looks so inviting with its layers of homemade granola, plant-based yogurt, and vivid raspberries. The recipe's natural sugars are balanced by the healthy fats, plant protein, and fiber-rich goodness. It's a picture-perfect, antioxidant-packed meal full of texture, taste, and satisfaction.

SERVES: 4 | SERVING SIZE: 1 jar
PREP TIME: 15 minutes | COOK TIME: 25 minutes

- 1½ cups old-fashioned, whole-grain rolled oats
- ⅓ cup slivered almonds
- 3 tablespoons raw wheat germ
- 2 tablespoons unsalted, shelled sunflower seeds or pepitas
- 2 teaspoons ground cinnamon
- 2 tablespoons natural, unsweetened apple butter
- 1½ tablespoons coconut nectar or date syrup
- 1⅓ cups plain, unsweetened, plant-based, Greek-style yogurt
- 1⅓ cups fresh raspberries

DIRECTIONS

1. Preheat the oven to 325°F. In a medium bowl, stir together the oats, almonds, wheat germ, sunflower seeds, and cinnamon.
2. In a small bowl, stir together the apple butter and coconut nectar. Add to the oat mixture and stir until thoroughly combined.
3. Spread the mixture evenly in a large baking pan. Bake until toasted and nearly crisp, about 25 minutes, stirring occasionally. Remove from the oven and let cool slightly to further crisp.
4. Layer the granola, plant-based yogurt, and raspberries into four jars, dessert bowls, or sundae glasses, and serve.

NUTRITION INFO

Choices/Exchanges: 2 starch, 1 carbohydrate, 1 medium fat protein, 1½ fat

Per serving: 340 calories, 12 g total fat, 1 g saturated fat, 0 g trans fat, 0 mg cholesterol, 80 mg sodium, 473 mg potassium, 44 g total carbohydrate, 9 g dietary fiber, 11 g sugars, 6 g added sugars, 16 g protein, 243 mg phosphorus

Say "Yes" to Oats

Whole oats are whole-grains that contain soluble (or viscous) fiber, which can help reduce blood cholesterol levels. And, in large quantities, soluble fiber may improve blood glucose control. That doesn't mean you can eat "super-sized" granola-raspberry jars! But it does mean it's a good idea to routinely include oats and oatmeal in your eating plan.

A Faster Fix

You can prepare the granola in this recipe ahead of time and store it in an airtight container at room temperature for several days. And instead of taking the time to layer it here as a parfait, simply dollop all the recipe ingredients into a bowl.

NO-BAKE BREAKFAST ENERGY BITES

When you don't have time for a sit-down breakfast, you'll love this fast and fun way to start the day. Make these tasty, button-shaped energy bites in advance and keep them chilled in the fridge so they're ready to go when you're on the go. (Hint: Have just two or three of them for an awesome energy boost at snack time, or for fueling up pre- or post-workout.)

SERVES: 3 | SERVING SIZE: 4 bites
PREP TIME: 18 minutes | COOK TIME: 0 minutes

- 12 pitted dates (the moister the better)
- 3 tablespoons creamy, natural, no-sugar-added peanut or pistachio butter
- ¼ teaspoon pure vanilla extract
- ⅛ teaspoon pure almond extract
- ⅛ teaspoon ground cinnamon
- ⅛ teaspoon sea salt
- ¼ cup old-fashioned, whole-grain rolled oats
- ¼ cup no-sugar-added puffed or crisp brown rice cereal
- ¼ cup salted, roasted peanuts
- 2 tablespoons sliced natural almonds or unsalted, shelled pistachios

DIRECTIONS

1. In a food processor, blend together all ingredients until a slightly textured dough forms.
2. Form into 12 buttons by extra-firmly packing mixture into a measuring tablespoon or a small cookie scoop. Or form into 1 tablespoon balls by hand. Ideally keep them chilled until ready to serve.

NUTRITION INFO

Choices/Exchanges: 2 fruit, 1 high fat protein, 2 fat

Per serving: 280 calories, 17 g total fat, 2.5 g saturated fat, 0 g trans fat, 0 mg cholesterol, 150 mg sodium, 393 mg potassium, 29 g total carbohydrate, 5 g dietary fiber, 20 g sugars, 0 g added sugars, 9 g protein, 82 mg phosphorus

Recipe Hints

After blending in the food processor, the dough mixture should stick together when firmly pressed between your thumb and first finger. If it doesn't, it may mean that your dates weren't moist. There's a fix for that: add more peanut butter by the teaspoon to reach desired texture.

Are Dates Good for You?

Sure, it can be healthy to go out on dates! But, if you're wondering about the type of dates that you actually eat, the answer is still yes. They provide fiber, a variety of antioxidants, and anti-inflammatory compounds. Studies suggest they may be associated with a neutral effect on A1C levels and potentially a beneficial impact on glycemic control for people with diabetes.

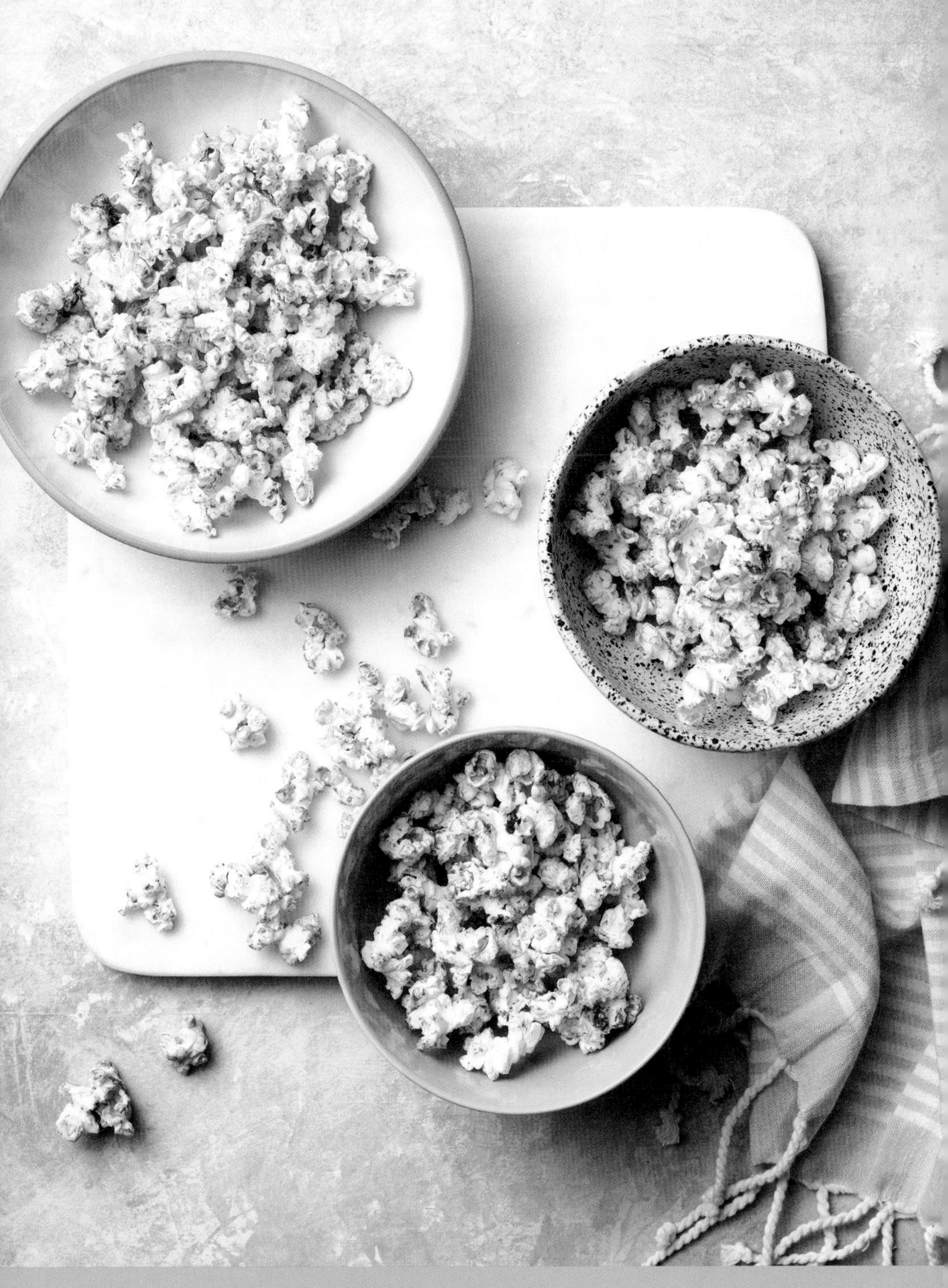

BBQ Stovetop Popcorn

Page 57

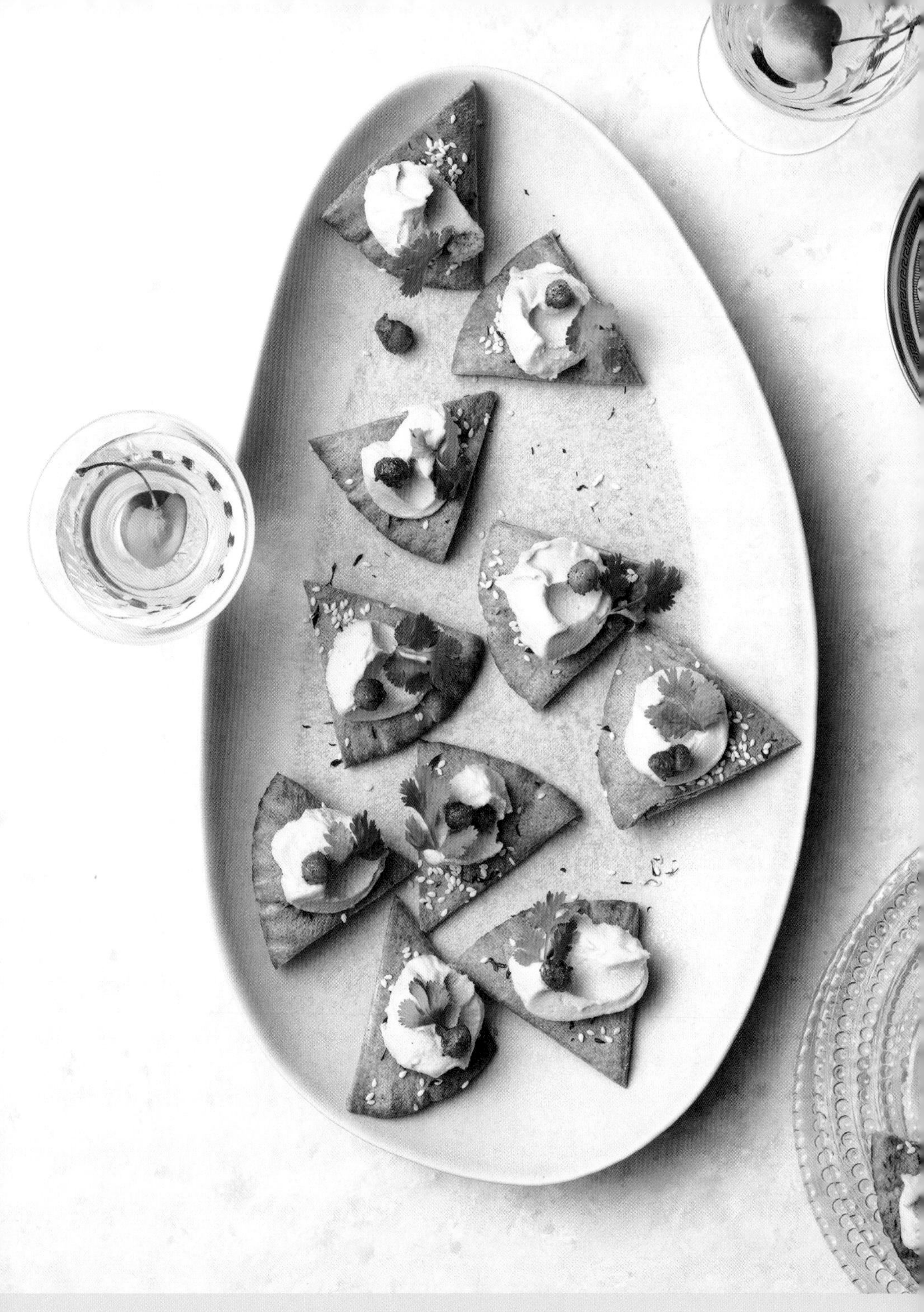

Party Hummus Canapés

Page 59

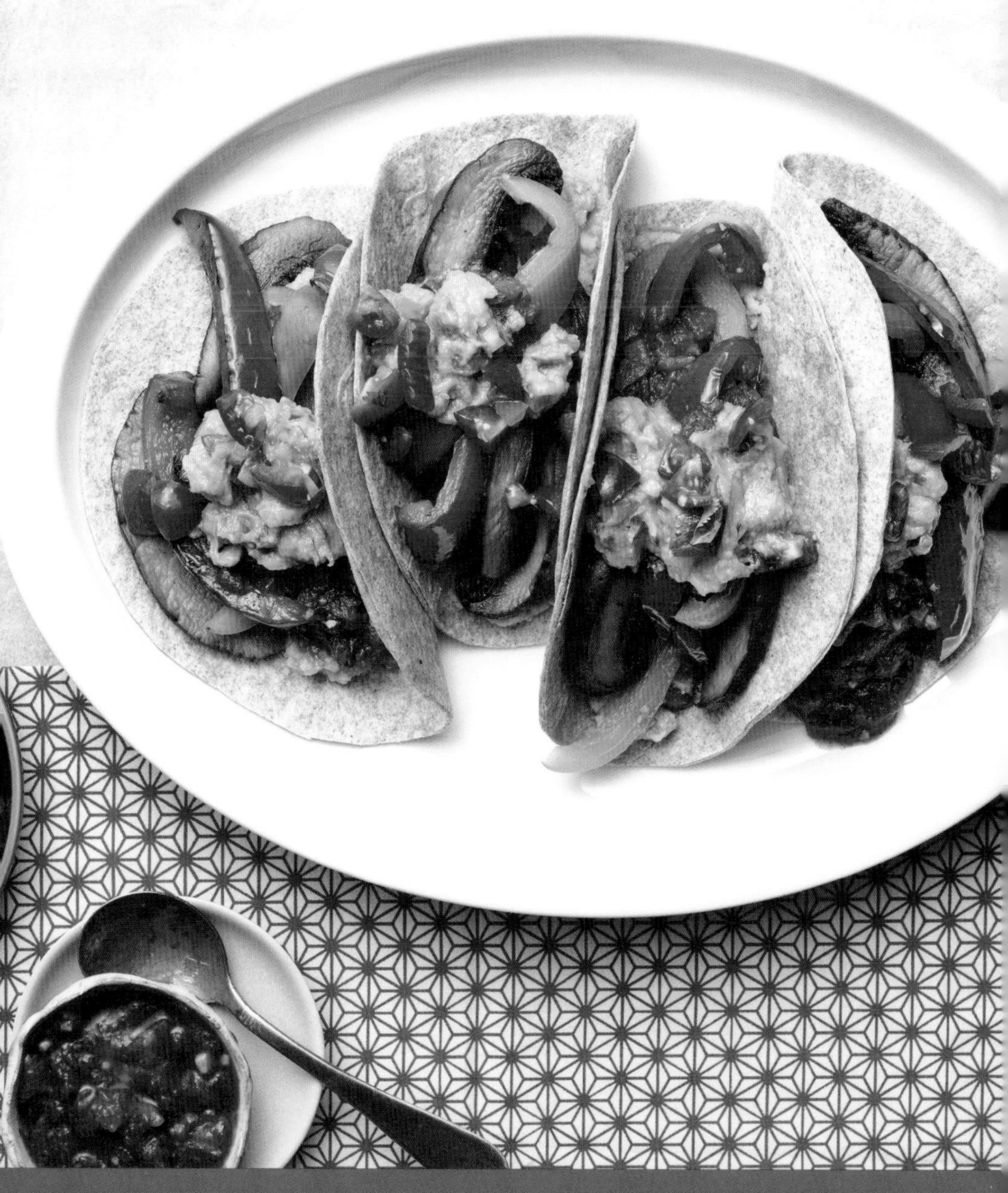

Portabella "Steak" Fajitas

Page 87

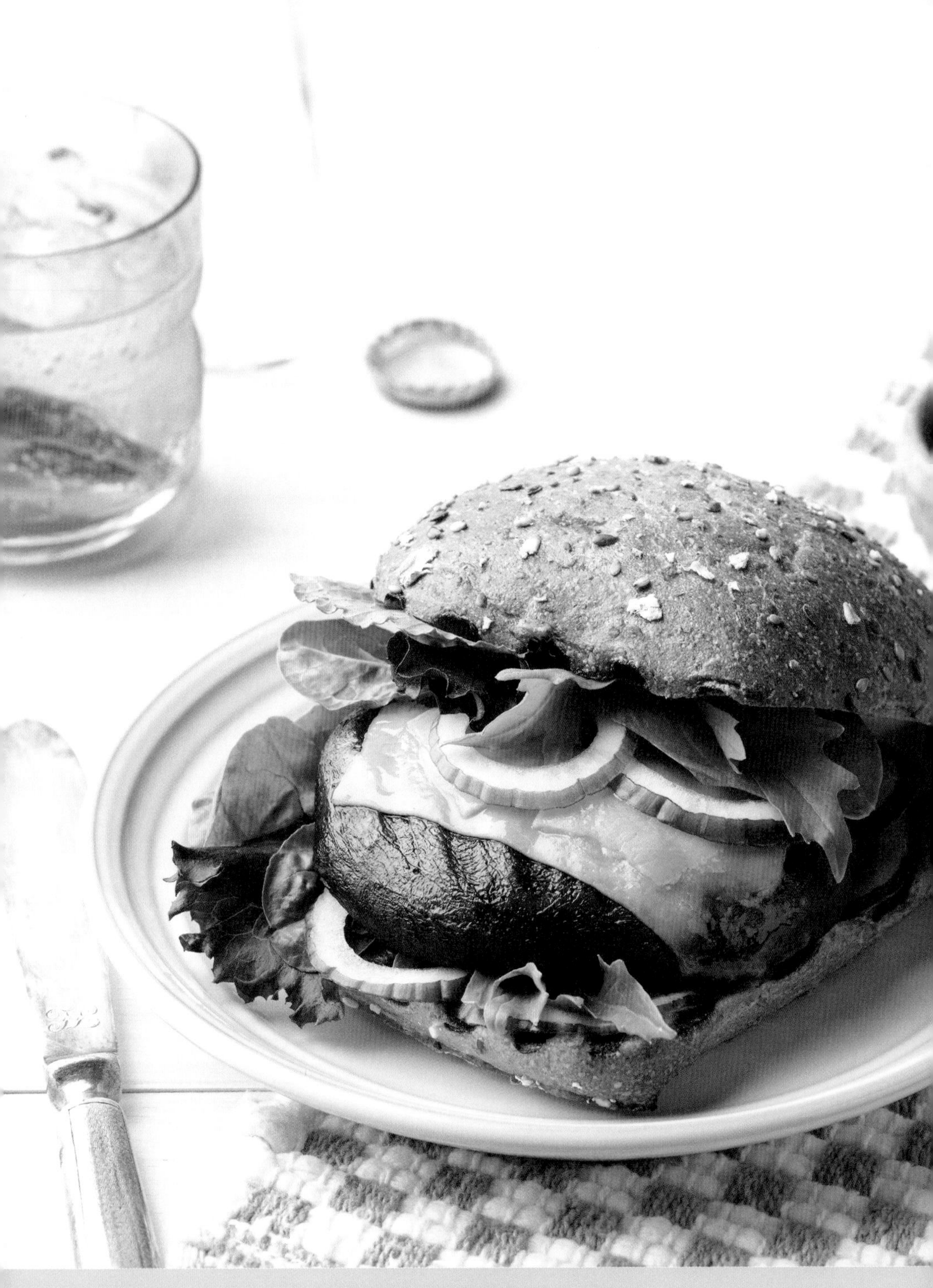

All-American Portabella Cheeseburgers

Page 125

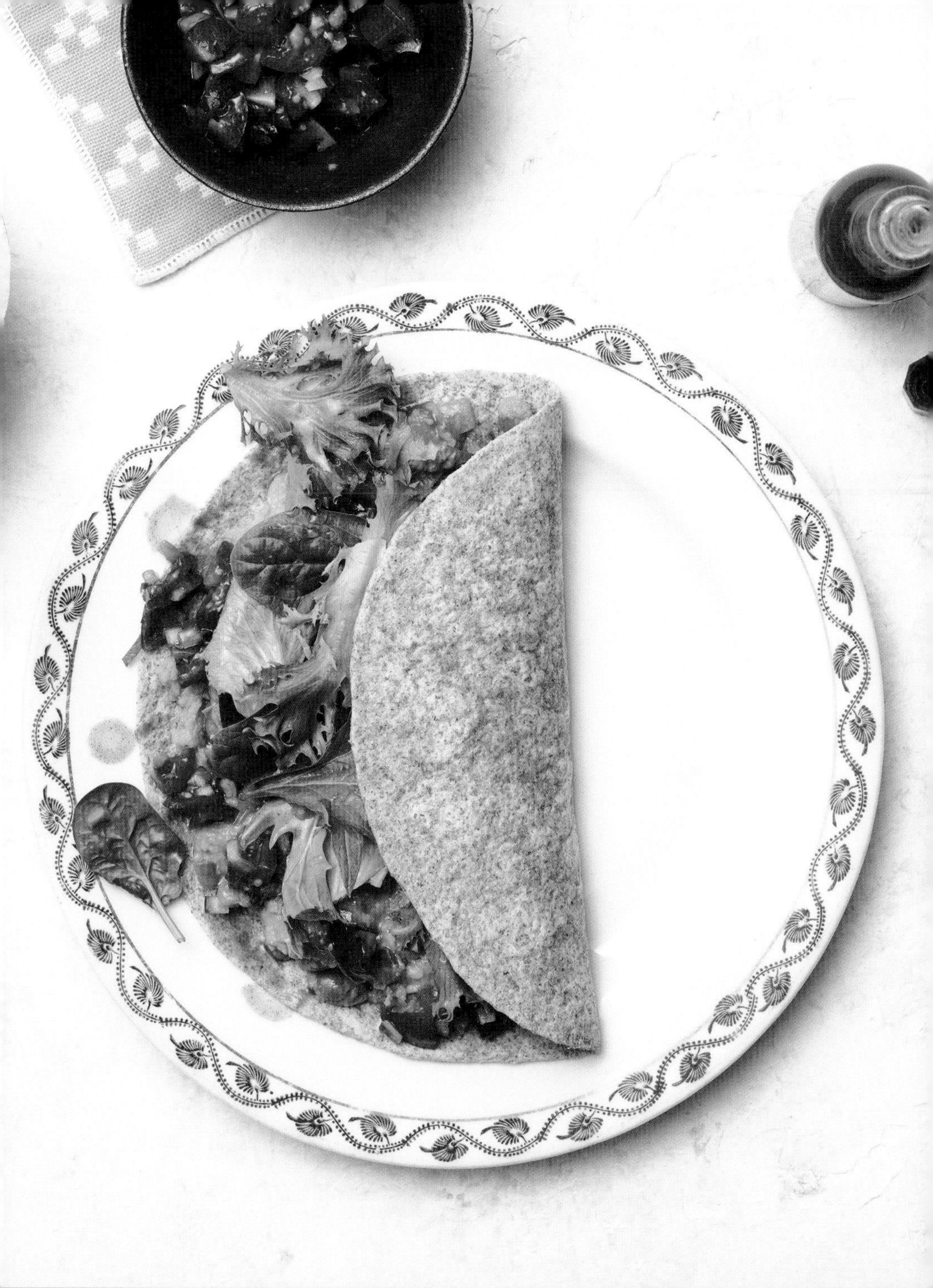

No-Brainer Bean Burrito Wrap

Page 141

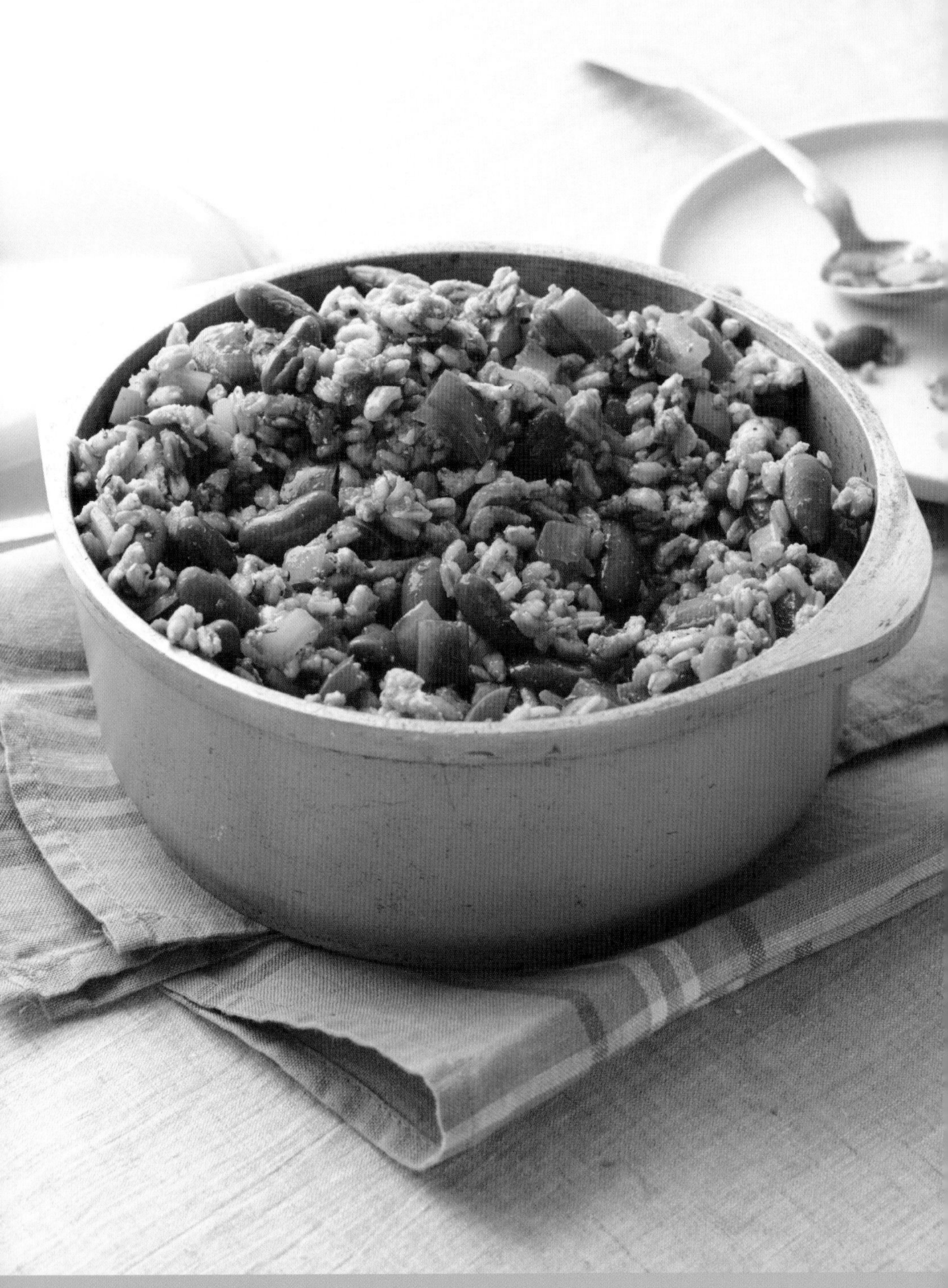

Cajan Grain Mini-Bowl

Page 165

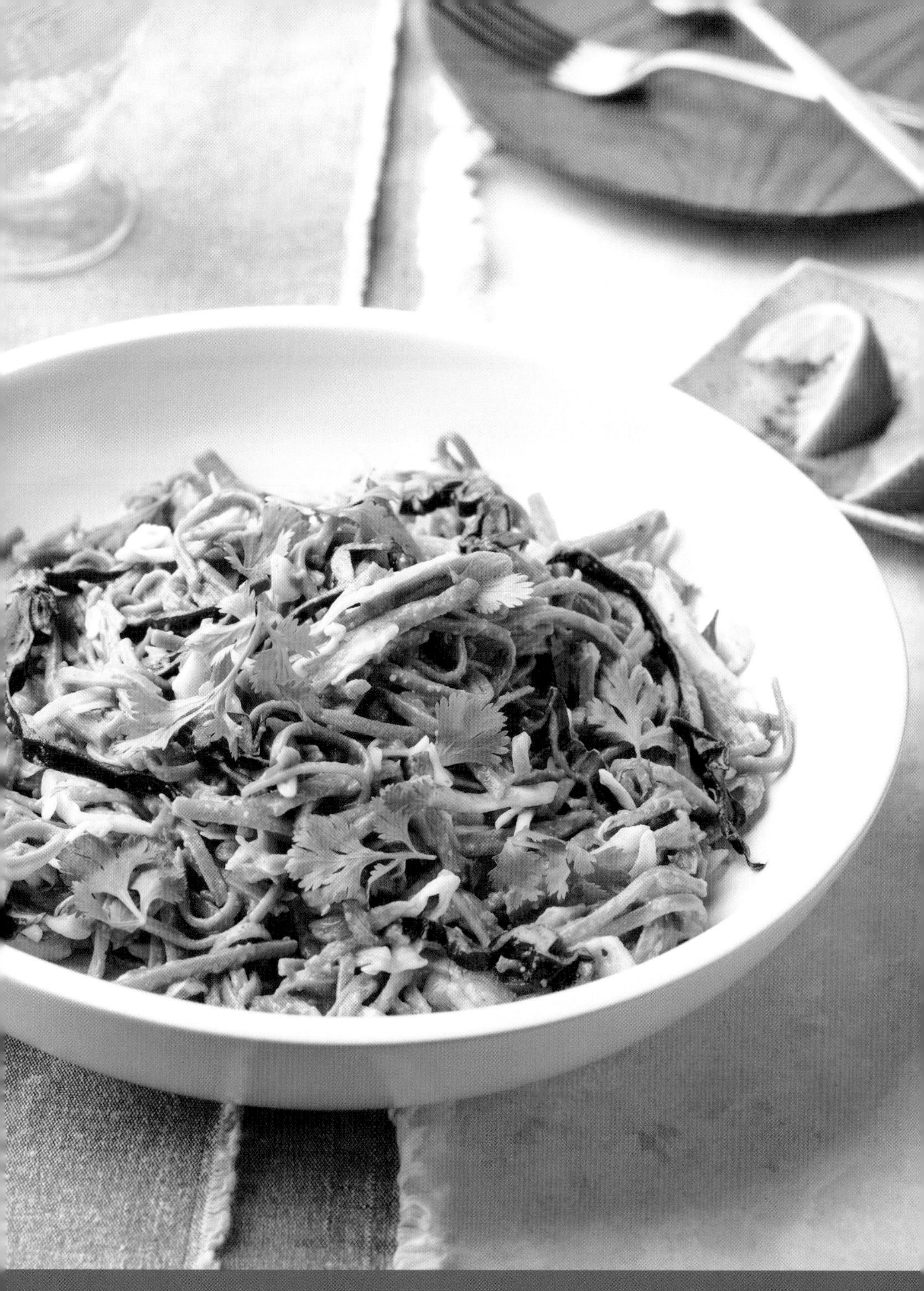

Saucy Peanut Soba Noodles with Slaw

Page 167

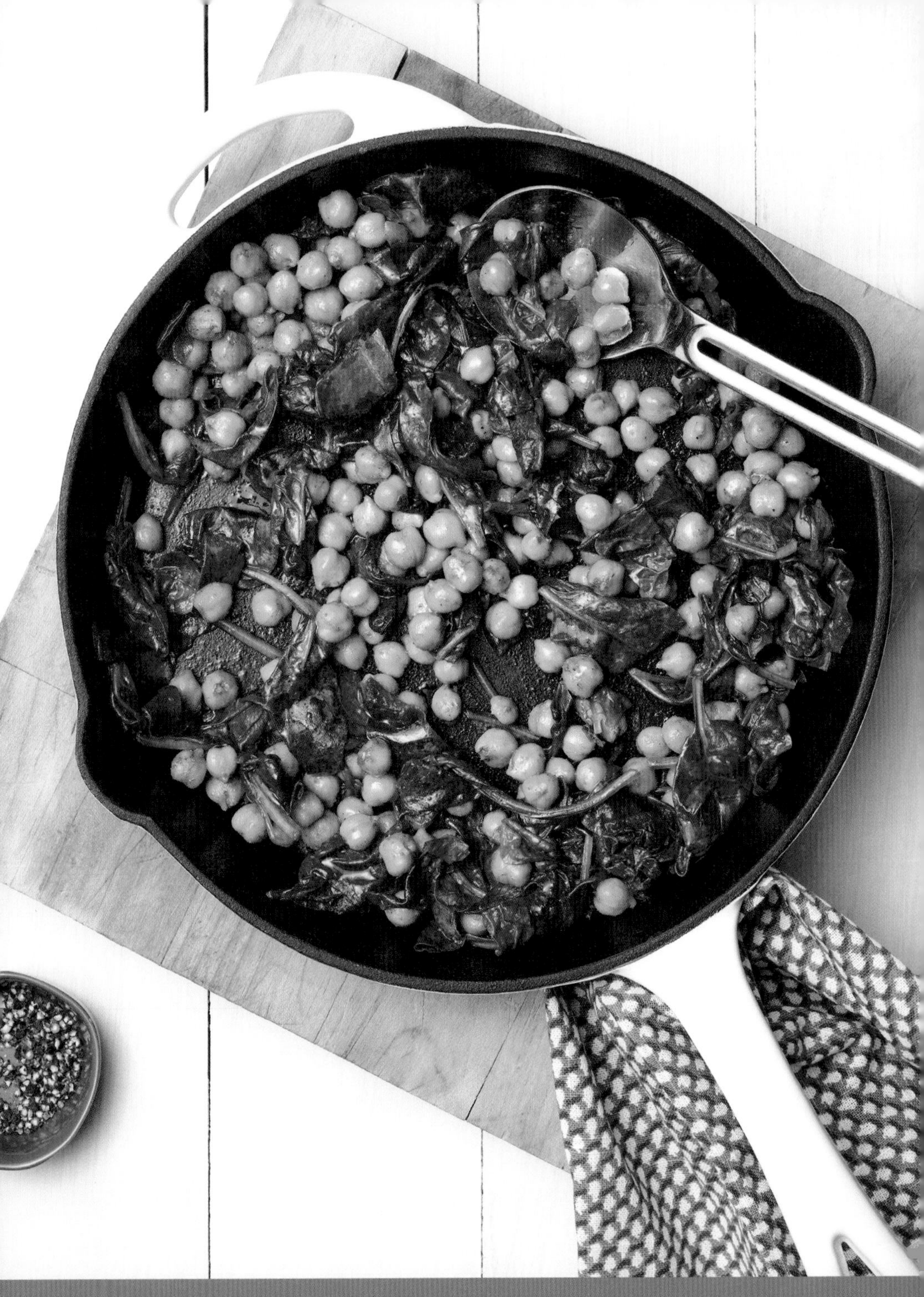

Skillet Beans and Greens with Coconutty Riced Cauliflower

Page 169

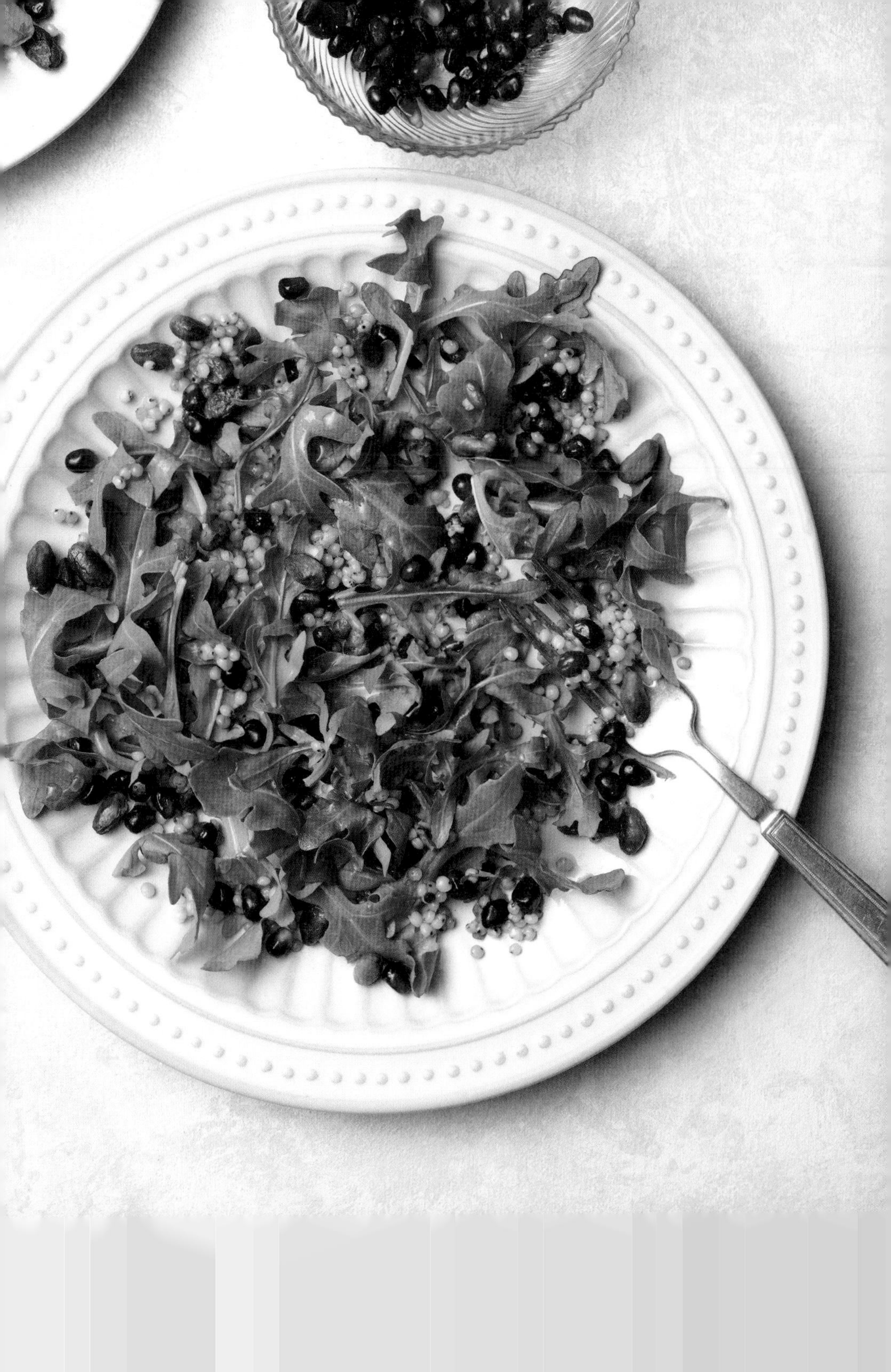

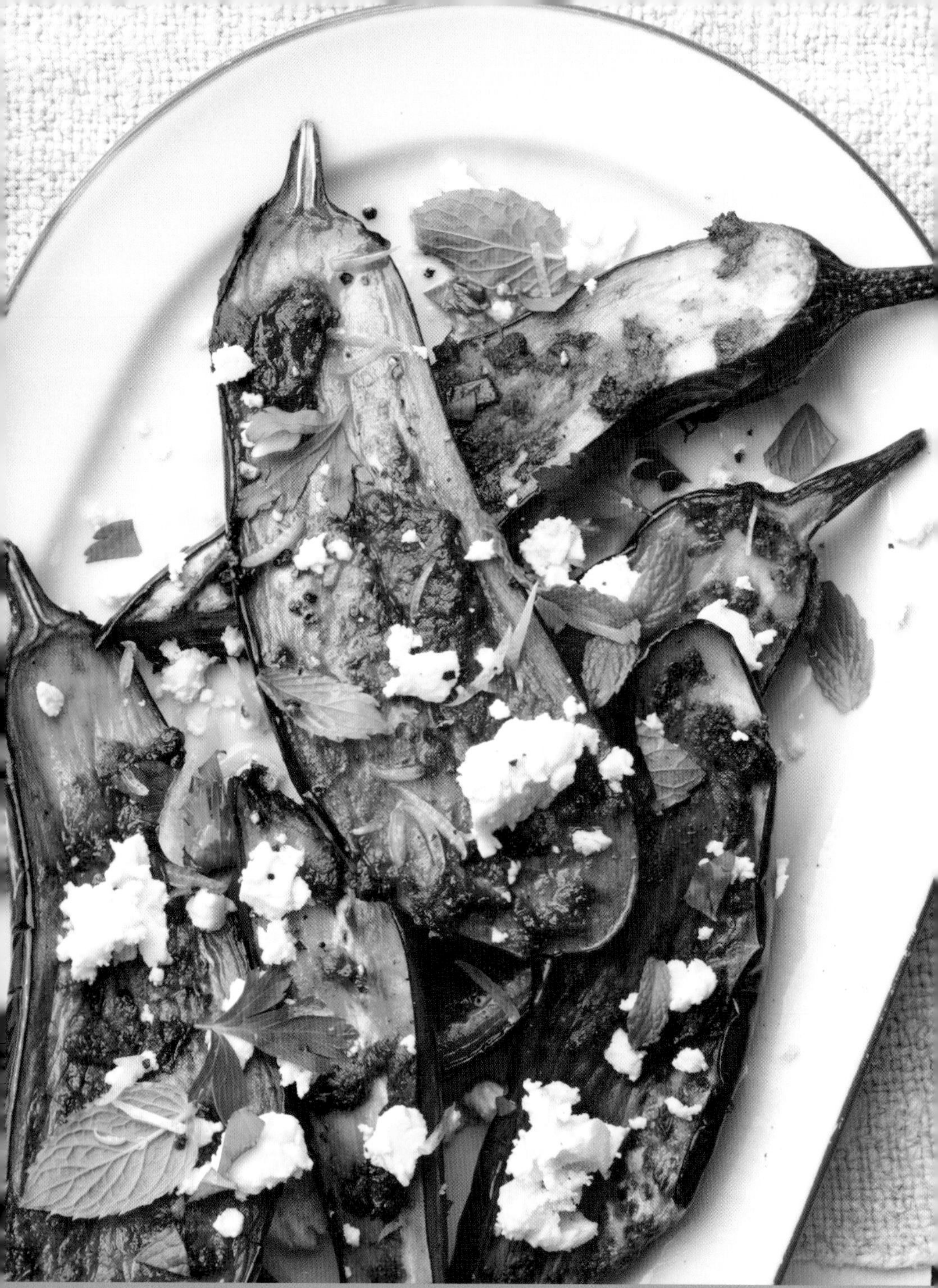

Roasted Greek Eggplant with Plant-Based Feta

Page 219

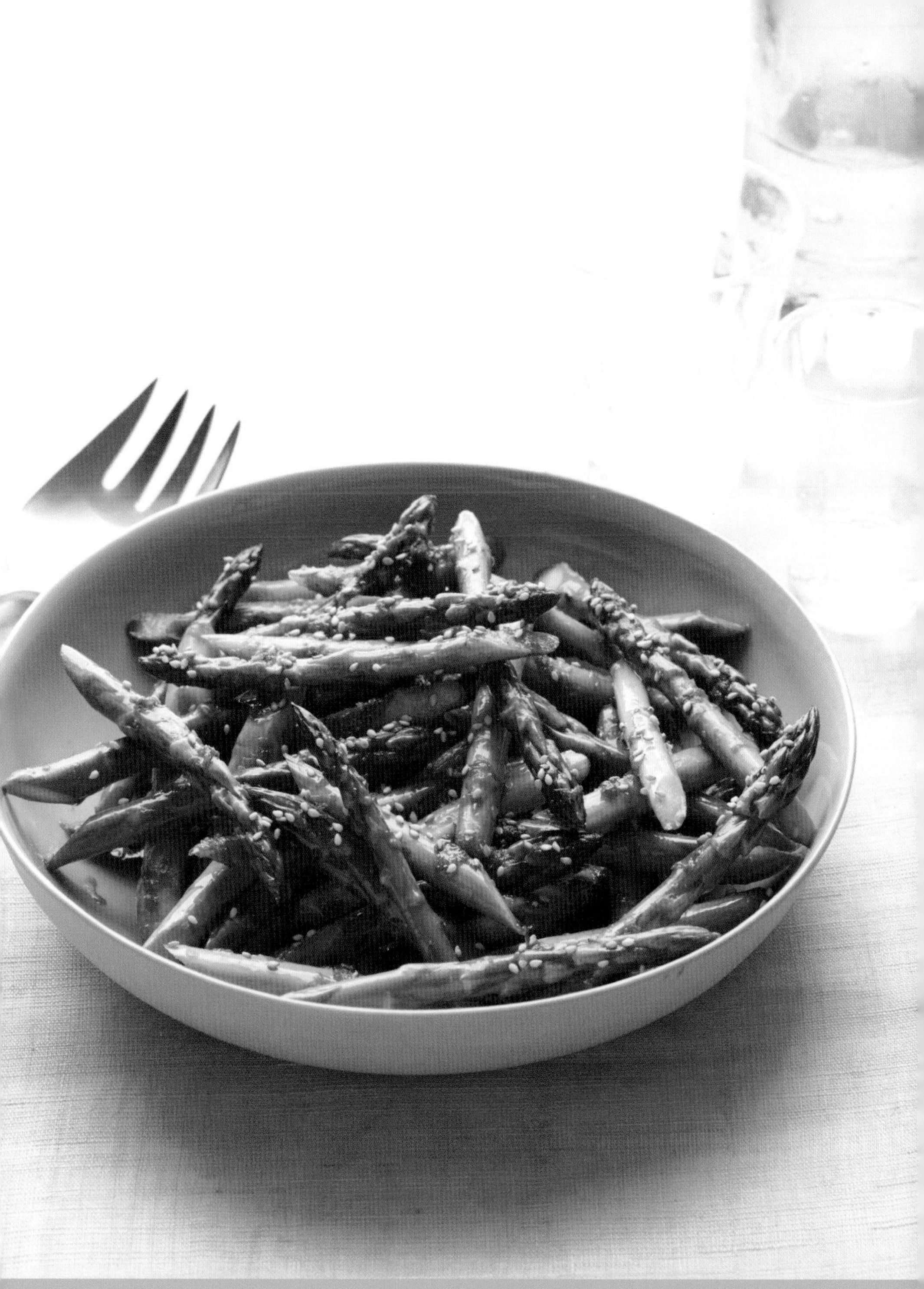

Spring Asparagus Stir-Fry

Page 225

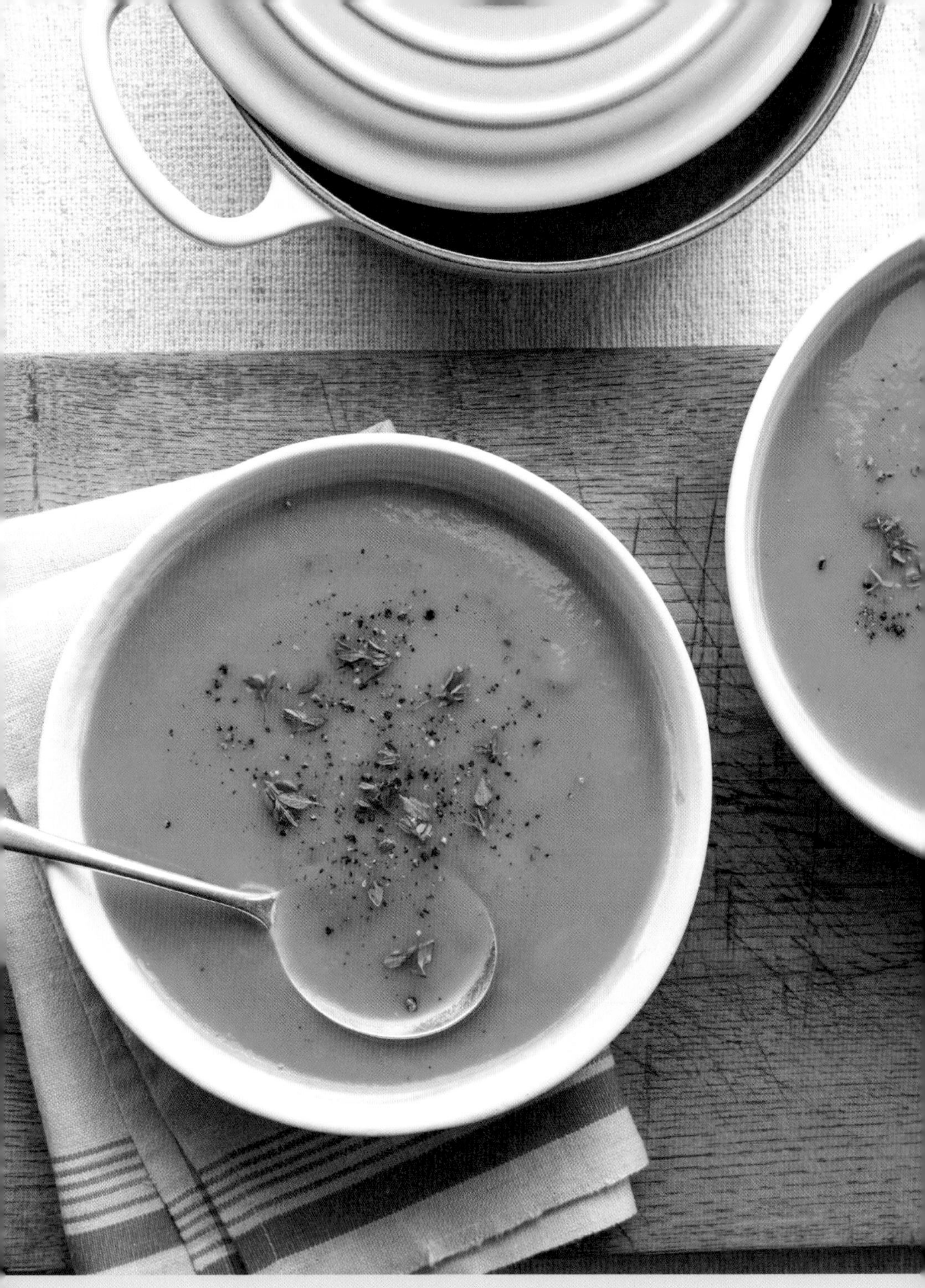

Roasted Orange Bell Pepper Soup

Page 247

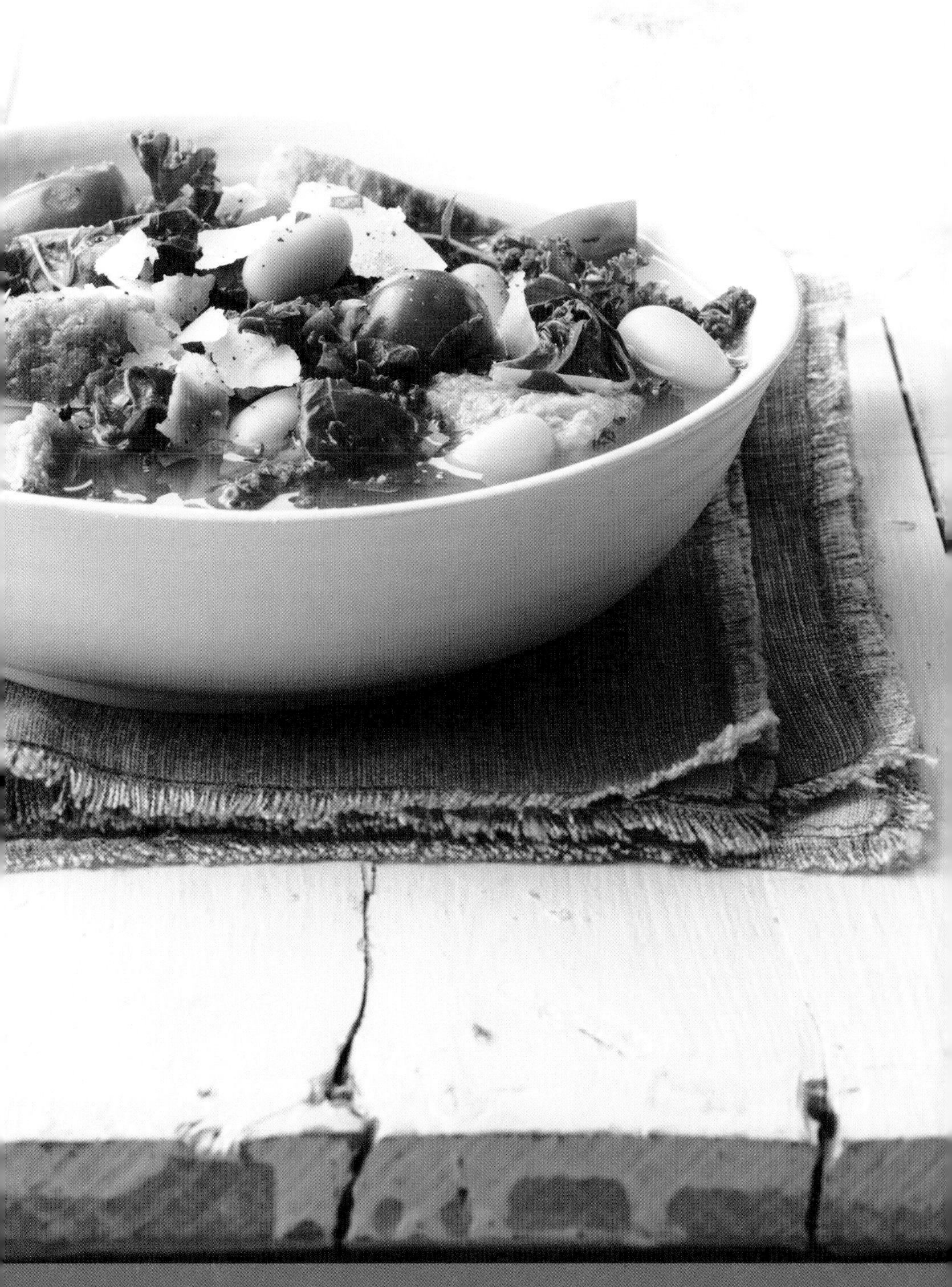

Tuscan Vegetable Stew

Page 255

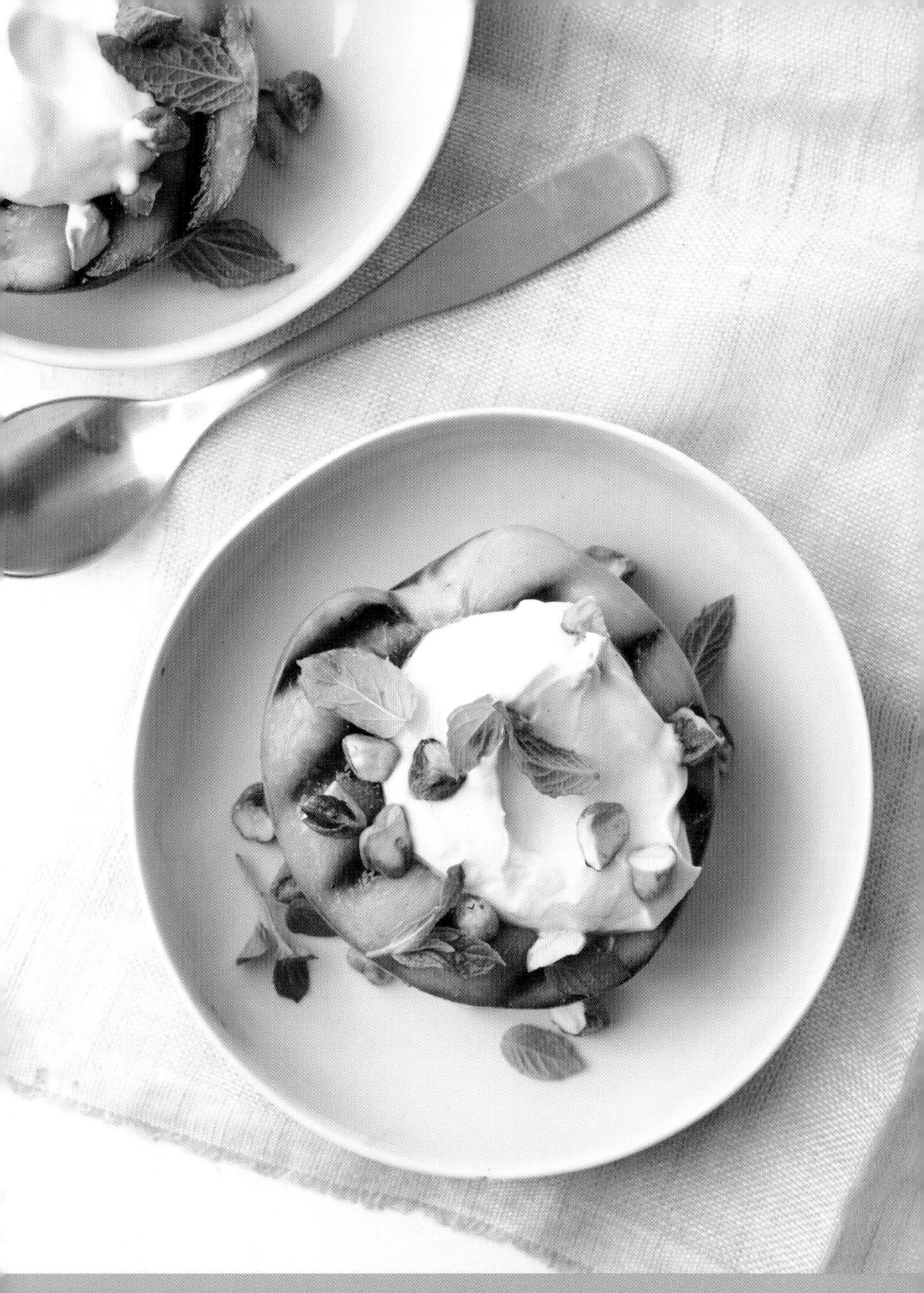

Just Peachy Bowls

Page 263

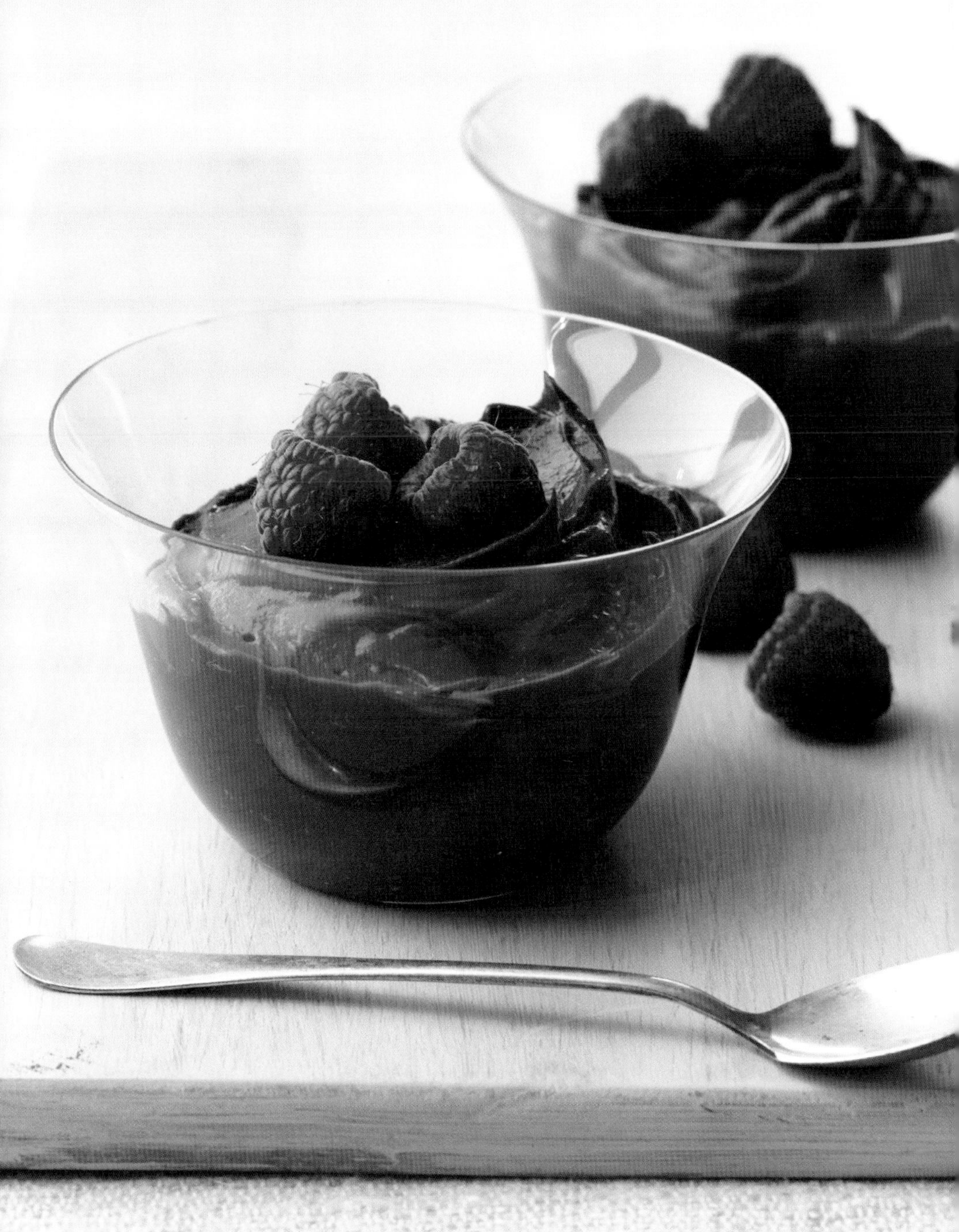

Dark Chocolate Raspberry Pudding

Page 265

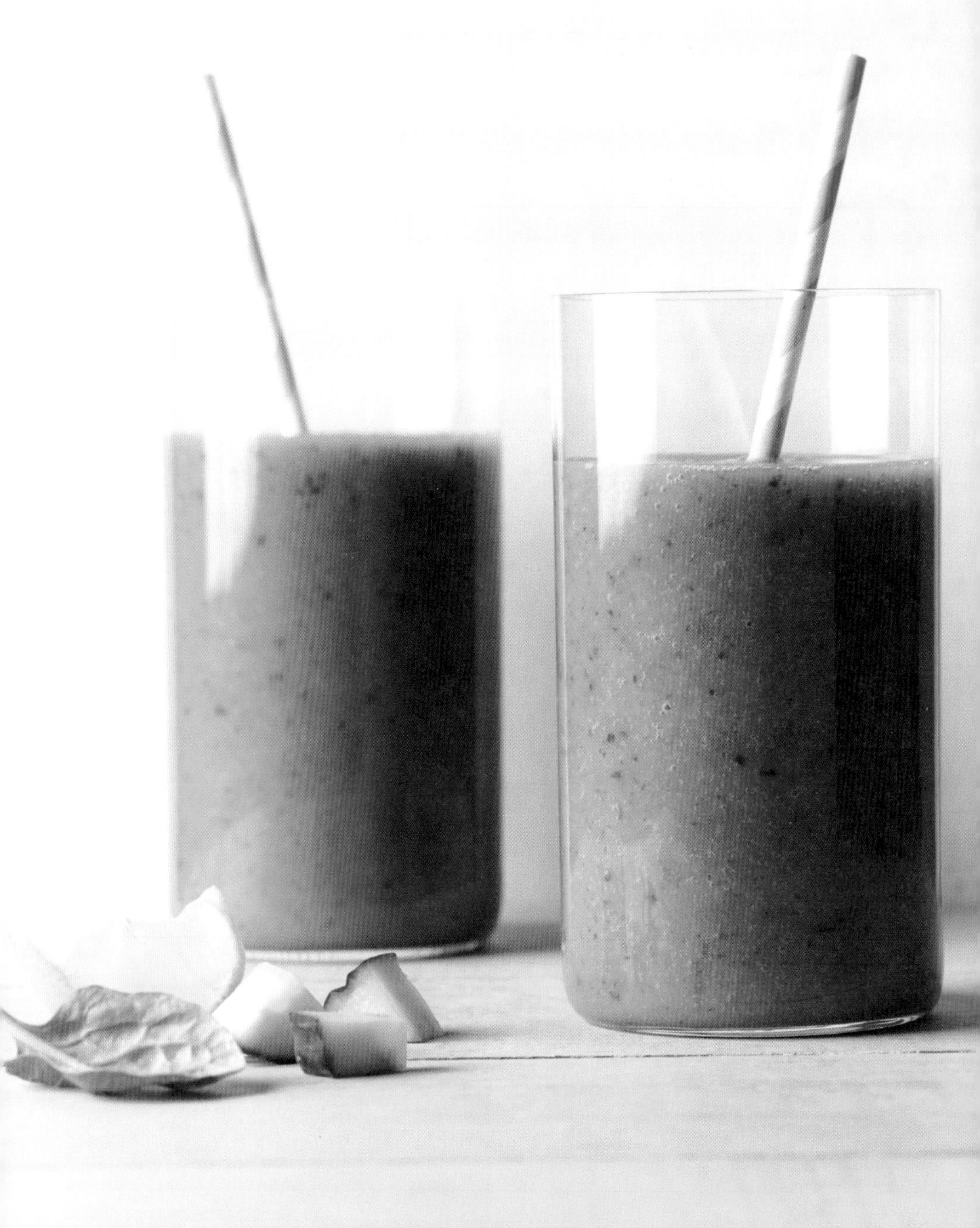

Green Juice Smoothie

Page 280

Main Dishes: Lunches and Dinners

PORTABELLA "STEAK" FAJITAS

The "steak" in these fajitas is free of beef thanks to meaty portabella mushroom caps. They provide an ideal heartiness here. To arrange your "steak" fajitas, try this: Spread each tortilla with the refried beans, top with the vegetable mixture and salsa, then add a dollop of guacamole. (Hint: I actually go a bit heavier on the guac for myself—so if your eating plan allows, go for it!) For a complete meal with Mexican appeal and more protein power, serve your fajitas with extra beans, like *Southwestern Cilantro-Lime Pintos* (page 209), on the side. This recipe can easily be doubled to feed a family of four—or you and three friends!

SERVES: 2 | SERVING SIZE: 2 fajitas
PREP TIME: 10 minutes | COOK TIME: 8 minutes

- 1 teaspoon avocado oil or peanut oil
- 2 large portabella mushrooms, stems removed, cut into ⅓-inch-wide slices
- 1 large green or red bell pepper (or half of each), cut into ⅓-inch-wide slices
- ¼ cup canned, lower-sodium, vegetarian refried beans
- 4 (5-inch) soft whole-wheat flour tortillas (about 1 ounce each)

- ¼ cup chunky preservative-free salsa or salsa verde
- ¼ cup guacamole of choice, or as desired (see recipes in this book)

DIRECTIONS

1. Heat the oil in a large cast-iron or other stick-resistant skillet over medium-high heat. Add the mushroom and bell pepper slices, and cook while tossing with tongs occasionally until the mushrooms are wilted and peppers are browned, about 8 minutes.
2. Meanwhile, add the refried beans to a small microwave-safe bowl. Heat in the microwave on high until hot, about 30 seconds.
3. Serve the vegetables (from the skillet), refried beans, tortillas, salsa, and guacamole separately so each person can assemble their own fajitas. Use 1 tablespoon refried beans, ¼ of the vegetable mixture, 1 tablespoon salsa, and 1 tablespoon guacamole per fajita.

NUTRITION INFO

Choices/Exchanges: 2 starch, 2 vegetable, 2½ fat

Per serving: 320 calories, 13 g total fat, 3.5 g saturated fat, 0 g trans fat, 0 mg cholesterol, 500 mg sodium, 940 mg potassium, 43 g total carbohydrate, 11 g dietary fiber, 7 g sugars, 0 g added sugars, 10 g protein, 340 mg phosphorus

Gills Are Good

You don't need to remove the portabella mushroom gills; they're 100 percent edible! But if you're weirded out by them, you can choose to scrape them out of the caps with a spoon.

Portabella Mushroom Stem Prep

If your portabella mushrooms have stems, snap them off by hand. Cook and savor them. For instance, thinly slice the stems into extra-thin coins, sauté in a little oil, and toss them into a pasta dish or serve as an avocado toast topper. Or season the sautéed slices with a pinch of smoked paprika, garlic powder, and sea salt, then enjoy as "pepperoni" for vegan pizza!

FAMILY-STYLE BB AND B FAJITAS

When are B's better than A's? When you're making this recipe! The three B's in the recipe title are for the savory stars you'll enjoy—beans, bell peppers, and broccoli. But the title isn't the only thing fun about these fajitas! Everyone gets to fill up their own tortilla in do-it-yourself (DIY) style. Your tortilla will be kind of stuffed, so you can wrap it up and eat burrito style if you prefer to keep it neat. And, if you're an avocado fanatic like me, it's okay to sneak in more guacamole. I won't tell; just plan for it!

SERVES: 6 | SERVING SIZE: 1 fajita
PREP TIME: 20 minutes | COOK TIME: 7 minutes

- ½ cup plain, unsweetened, plant-based Greek-style yogurt
- 2 tablespoons chopped fresh cilantro
- Juice of ½ lime (1 tablespoon), divided
- 1 (15-ounce) can pinto or black beans, gently rinsed and drained (1½ cups)
- ⅔ cup *Grape Tomato Pico de Gallo* (page 142) or deli-prepared pico de gallo
- 1 tablespoon peanut or avocado oil
- 1 medium white onion, halved, sliced
- 1 small jalapeño pepper with some seeds, halved lengthwise and thinly sliced crosswise
- 2 large red or green bell peppers, or one of each, thinly sliced
- 2 cups broccoli slaw (shredded mixture of broccoli, carrots and red cabbage)
- ½ teaspoon ground cumin, or to taste
- ¼ teaspoon sea salt, or to taste
- ½ cup guacamole of choice, or as desired (recipes in book and as follows)
- 6 soft taco-size whole-wheat or other tortillas

DIRECTIONS

1. Stir together the plant-based yogurt, cilantro, and 1 teaspoon of the lime juice in a small bowl and set aside.
2. Stir together the beans and pico de gallo in a small saucepan. Cover and place over low heat to warm.
3. Meanwhile, heat the oil in a wok or large deep skillet over medium-high heat. Add the onion and jalapeño and sauté until the onion is slightly softened, about 2 minutes. Increase heat to high, add the bell peppers, broccoli slaw, cumin, salt, and the remaining 2 teaspoons lime juice, and stir-fry until all vegetables are cooked through and the onion is lightly caramelized, about 4 minutes. Transfer to a serving dish and adjust seasoning.
4. Serve the vegetable mixture (4 cups), bean mixture (2 cups), yogurt mixture (⅔ cup), and guacamole (½ cup) family style with the tortillas.

NUTRITION INFO

Choices/Exchanges: 2 starch, 1 vegetable, 2 fat

Per serving: 270 calories, 10 g total fat, 2 g saturated fat, 0 g trans fat, 0 mg cholesterol, 550 mg sodium, 517 mg potassium, 36 g total carbohydrate, 7 g dietary fiber, 6 g sugars, 0 g added sugars, 10 g protein, 77 mg phosphorus

JACKIE'S HASS AVOCADO GUACAMOLE

- 1 Hass avocado, pitted, peeled, and cubed
- 2 teaspoons fresh lime juice
- 2 to 3 tablespoons diced red onion, or to taste
- 1 tablespoon chopped fresh cilantro
- ½ small jalapeño pepper, with some seeds, minced
- ¼ teaspoon ground coriander
- ¼ teaspoon sea salt, or to taste

DIRECTIONS

Stir together all of the ingredients in a medium bowl until combined, and serve. (Makes ¾ cup; 6 servings, 2 tablespoons each.)

NUTRITION INFO

Choices/Exchanges: 1 fat

Per serving: 40 calories, 3.5 g total fat, 0.5 g saturated fat, 0 g trans fat, 0 mg cholesterol, 100 mg sodium, 130 mg potassium, 3 g total carbohydrate, 2 g dietary fiber, 0 g sugars, 0 g added sugars, 1 g protein, 10 mg phosphorus

KUNG PAO TOFU AND PEPPERS

This Kung Pao sure packs a pow. Typically based on chicken, this plant-based take on the popular Chinese stir-fry dish is rich in color, texture, and flavor. The Asian-flavored baked tofu makes it a bona fide entrée. And the peanuts and peppers are still key features. But the best part for some may be that once you prep the ingredients, it takes just 5 minutes from wok to table. Enjoy over buckwheat soba noodles or steamed brown rice. Serve soy sauce with a splash of rice vinegar on the side for additional pep, if you like.

SERVES: 4 | SERVING SIZE: 1¼ cups
PREP TIME: 18 minutes | COOK TIME: 5 minutes

- 1 tablespoon avocado oil or peanut oil
- 3 large bell peppers, various colors, diced
- 1 small serrano pepper with some seeds, thinly sliced
- 1 tablespoon freshly grated gingerroot
- 3 large garlic cloves, very thinly sliced
- ¾ cup *Simple Stir-Fry Sauce* (recipe follows)
- 4 scallions, green and white parts, sliced diagonally
- 3 tablespoons coarsely chopped, salted, dry-roasted peanuts
- 6 ounces Asian-flavored (or sesame ginger) ready-to-eat baked organic tofu, diced

DIRECTIONS

1. Heat the oil in a wok or large deep skillet over high heat. Carefully add the bell peppers, serrano pepper, ginger, and garlic and stir-fry until the bell peppers are *al dente*, about 3 minutes. Add the stir-fry sauce and scallions and stir-fry until the sauce is slightly thickened, about 30 seconds. Add the peanuts and stir-fry until the sauce is thickened, about 30 seconds.
2. Immediately stir in the tofu until heated through, about 30 seconds, and serve.

NUTRITION INFO

Choices/Exchanges: 2 vegetable, 1 medium fat protein, 2 fat

Per serving: 230 calories, 14 g total fat, 2 g saturated fat, 0 g trans fat, 0 mg cholesterol, 460 mg sodium, 500 mg potassium, 16 g total carbohydrate, 4 g dietary fiber, 6 g sugars, 0 g added sugars, 14 g protein, 200 mg phosphorus

SIMPLE STIR-FRY SAUCE

- ½ cup low-sodium vegetable broth
- 2 tablespoons unsweetened applesauce
- 1 tablespoon rice or brown rice vinegar
- 1 tablespoon naturally brewed soy sauce
- 1½ teaspoons toasted sesame oil
- 2 teaspoons organic cornstarch

Whisk together the broth, applesauce, vinegar, soy sauce, oil, and cornstarch in a liquid measuring cup until smooth. (Makes ¾ cup; 4 servings, 3 tablespoons each.)

NUTRITION INFO
Choices/Exchanges: ½ fat
Per serving: 30 calories, 2 g total fat, 0 g saturated fat, 0 g trans fat, 250 mg sodium, 10 mg potassium, 3 g total carbohydrate, 0 g dietary fiber, 1 g sugars, 0 g added sugars, 1 g protein, 0 mg phosphorus

CREAMY VEGAN EGGPLANT KORMA

If you're in the mood for tasty comfort food, this recipe is made for you. It has distinct Indian cuisine flavors but is balanced enough for nearly every palate. The creamy korma is full of wonderful textures, including crunchiness from the almonds, along with pops of color from the tomato and cilantro. You'll love how the tomatoes burst in your mouth. Enjoy it as is or served over steamed brown basmati rice or whole-wheat couscous.

SERVES: 4 | SERVING SIZE: 1¾ cups
PREP TIME: 22 minutes | COOK TIME: 33 minutes

- 2 teaspoons avocado oil or unrefined peanut oil
- 1 medium red onion, finely diced
- 1 (15-ounce) can no-salt-added tomato sauce, divided
- ½ teaspoon sea salt, divided
- 1 large (1½-pound) eggplant, unpeeled, cut into ½-inch cubes
- 3 large garlic cloves, minced
- 2 teaspoons freshly grated gingerroot
- 2 tablespoons creamy, natural, no-sugar-added peanut or almond butter
- 1 tablespoon garam masala curry paste or other red curry paste
- 2 teaspoons ground coriander
- ¼ cup finely chopped dried unsulfured apricots or black seedless raisins
- 1¼ cups plain, unsweetened, plant-based milk of choice, such as coconut milk beverage
- 1 pint grape tomatoes
- 3 tablespoons sliced natural almonds, pan-toasted
- ¼ cup chopped fresh cilantro

DIRECTIONS

1. Heat the oil in a large, deep, stick-resistant skillet or Dutch oven over medium heat. Add the onion, ¼ cup of the tomato sauce, and ¼ teaspoon of the salt and sauté until the onion is softened, about 8 minutes. Add the eggplant, garlic, and ginger, and cook while stirring until the eggplant is heated through, about 3 minutes.

2. Add the peanut butter, curry paste, coriander, and the remaining tomato sauce. Cook while stirring until the mixture is well-combined and steamy hot, about 5 minutes. Add the dried apricots, plant-based milk, and the remaining ¼ teaspoon salt and bring to a boil over high heat.
3. Reduce heat to medium-low and simmer, covered, until the eggplant is fully cooked, about 10 minutes, stirring a couple times during the simmering process. Stir in the grape tomatoes and simmer, covered, until the tomatoes are heated through, about 5 minutes. Adjust seasoning.
4. Ladle the korma into individual bowls, sprinkle with the almonds and cilantro, and serve.

NUTRITION INFO
Choices/Exchanges: 1 carbohydrate, 4 vegetable, 2 fat
Per serving: 240 calories, 10 g total fat, 1 g saturated fat, 0 g trans fat, 0 mg cholesterol, 490 mg sodium, 1090 mg potassium, 31 g total carbohydrate, 9 g dietary fiber, 18 g sugars, 0 g added sugars, 8 g protein, 150 mg phosphorus

Heart-Healthy Oil "Cheat Sheet"

In general, for a multipurpose oil, use avocado oil or high-oleic sunflower oil for their high smoke points and neutral flavors. They're fine for cooking or baking at all temps or for no cooking at all. For cooking on medium heat or lower, or for use on fresh dishes or to finish hot dishes, use extra-virgin olive oil when you desire its robust flavor. And when desiring their unique flavor profiles, use nut or seed oils, like toasted sesame oil. But know that these are not "rules," so go ahead and mix and match oils to recipes as you see fit.

EASY GINGER TEMPEH AND SNOW PEA STIR-FRY

Tempeh might look a bit odd, but it's just a fermented soybean cake . . . a savory cake! Its "meaty" texture works delightfully in this stir-fry, which features a simple yet highly flavored sauce made from only three ingredients—unsweetened applesauce, reduced-sodium tamari (soy sauce), and fresh gingerroot. You'll also use a cooking technique that's basically a "dry" stir-fry, so no excess sauce or oil is required, keeping its calories in check. This leaves room for you to pair it with steamed brown rice or other whole grains, and more.

SERVES: 2 I SERVING SIZE: 2 cups
PREP TIME: 15 minutes I COOK TIME: 8 minutes

- 2 teaspoons toasted sesame oil
- 8 ounces organic tempeh, halved lengthwise, then cut crosswise into thin (⅓-inch-wide) strips
- 2 cups fresh snow peas, ends trimmed (5 ounces)
- 3 scallions, green and white parts, cut into 1½-inch pieces
- ⅓ cup unsweetened applesauce
- 1 tablespoon + 1 teaspoon reduced-sodium tamari (soy sauce)
- 1½ teaspoons grated fresh gingerroot

DIRECTIONS

1. Heat the oil in a wok or large, deep skillet over medium-high heat. Add the tempeh and cook while stirring occasionally until the tempeh is golden brown, about 4 minutes. Add the snow peas and scallions, and cook while stirring until they begin to brown, about 3 minutes.
2. Stir in the applesauce, tamari, and ginger; remove from heat and serve.

NUTRITION INFO

Choices/Exchanges: ½ starch, ½ carbohydrate, 1 vegetable, 3 medium fat protein

Per serving: 320 calories, 17 g total fat, 3.6 g saturated fat, 0 g trans fat, 0 mg cholesterol, 340 mg sodium, 730 mg potassium, 21 g total carbohydrate, 3 g dietary fiber, 15 g sugars, 0 g added sugars, 26 g protein, 365 mg phosphorus

Recipe Variations

No snow peas? You can make this stir-fry with any non-starchy vegetable that you have on hand, like green beans, sliced bell peppers, chopped asparagus, or broccoli florets. Got calories to spare? Top with dry-roasted peanuts for crunch or with pan-toasted sesame seeds for intrigue. Want bonus flavor dazzle? Sprinkle with fresh cilantro leaves or hot sauce.

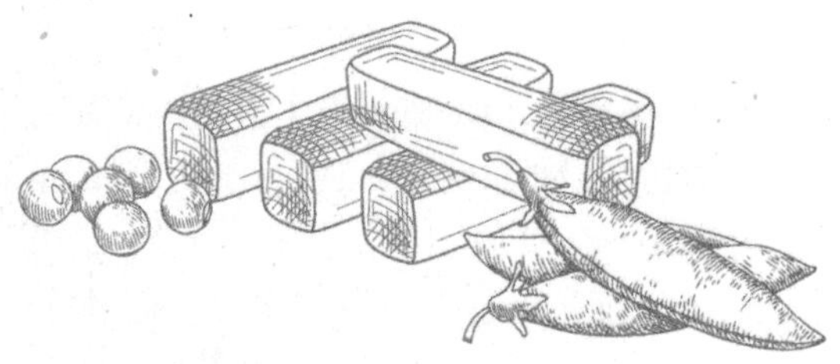

SIMPLE SPICE-RUBBED CAULIFLOWER ROAST

There's truly no sweat involved with this impressive entrée. It's spiced, not spicy! Make the cauliflower roast (yes, the whole head!) for a special occasion and serve half of it as the main dish for anyone—even meat eaters. Or go ahead and make any day special by roasting this on a regular weekday for anyone (yes, that includes you!). It's wow-worthy but so easy to make. Change up the spices from time to time to keep your palate enticed. Serve it with a protein-rich side, like *Zesty Mandarin Edamame* (page 211), to make it a substantial meal.

SERVES: 2 | SERVING SIZE: ½ cauliflower head
PREP TIME: 8 minutes | COOK TIME: 1 hour 40 minutes

- 1 large (2½-pound) head cauliflower
- 1 tablespoon extra-virgin olive oil
- 1 teaspoon curry powder
- ¾ teaspoon ground ginger
- ½ teaspoon freshly ground black pepper
- ¼ teaspoon sea salt

DIRECTIONS

1. Preheat the oven to 375°F.
2. Cut off enough of the cauliflower stem so that the head can stand upright. Then cut or snap off the outer leaves. Place the whole cauliflower onto a cast-iron skillet or a baking pan. Brush or rub the entire head with the oil.
3. In a small bowl, stir together the curry powder, ginger, pepper, and salt. Sprinkle or rub the cauliflower head with the spice mixture.
4. Cover the cauliflower well—including the pan—with foil. Roast for 1 hour. Remove foil and roast uncovered until cooked through and well caramelized, about 35–40 minutes more.
5. Cut in half or slice into "steaks." Serve.

NUTRITION INFO

Choices/Exchanges: 3 vegetable, 1½ fat

Per serving: 150 calories, 8 g total fat, 1.4 g saturated fat, 0 g trans fat, 0 mg cholesterol, 370 mg sodium, 1050 mg potassium, 18 g total carbohydrate, 7 g dietary fiber, 7 g sugars, 0 g added sugars, 7 g protein, 155 mg phosphorus

Spice Swaps

Cauliflower has a mild taste, yet pairs well with a variety of not-so-mild herbs and spices. For a change of taste, consider other global-cuisine-inspired options in place of the curry powder and ginger. Try ground cumin and ground cinnamon for a Lebanese spin, or dried tarragon and garlic powder for French flair.

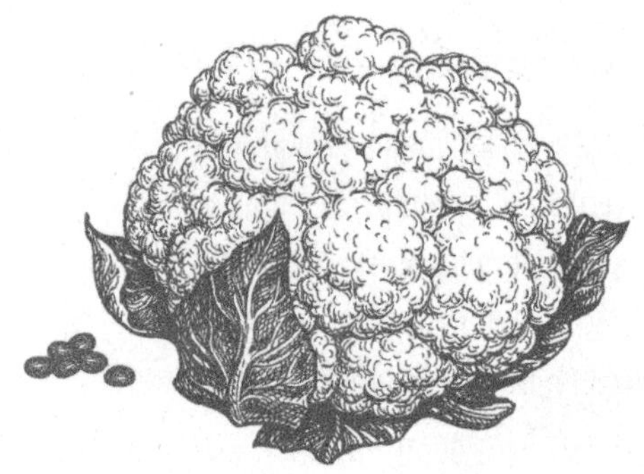

CARAMELIZED CAULIFLOWER AND HERBS ON BED OF HUMMUS

Hummus has a culinary life well beyond just as a popular snack dip. This recipe transforms the concept of hummus and veggies into a warm and comforting entrée featuring sautéed caramelized cauliflower. The toppings, including a sprinkling of hot pepper sauce, fresh herb sprigs, and pan-toasted pine nuts, create cuisine magic. When you can find it, use purple or golden cauliflower for bonus enticement. Complete the meal with whole-grain pita and a simple side salad. It's a surprising delight!

SERVES: 4 | SERVING SIZE: 2 cups
PREP TIME: 12 minutes | COOK TIME: 19 minutes

- 1¼ cups hummus of choice (see recipes in this book)
- 1 tablespoon extra-virgin olive oil
- 1½ pounds cauliflower florets (7 cups)*
- ⅛ teaspoon sea salt
- 1½ teaspoons hot pepper sauce, or to taste
- ½ cup small fresh parsley, mint, or cilantro sprigs
- 2 tablespoons pine nuts, pan-toasted

**Note: A large 2-pound head of cauliflower provides 1½ pounds florets.*

DIRECTIONS

1. Thinly spread 5 tablespoons (that's basically a rounded ¼ cup) hummus onto each of 4 luncheon-sized plates.
2. Fully heat the oil in a large, deep, cast-iron or other stick-resistant skillet over medium heat. Add the cauliflower florets and cook while stirring occasionally until cooked through and golden brown, about 18 minutes. Sprinkle with the salt.
3. Divide the cauliflower evenly among the 4 plates and arrange on top of the hummus. Drizzle each plate with the hot pepper sauce. Sprinkle each with parsley sprigs and ½ tablespoon pine nuts. Serve.

NUTRITION INFO

Choices/Exchanges: ½ starch, 2 vegetable, 1 medium fat protein, 1½ fat

Per serving: 230 calories, 14 g total fat, 2 g saturated fat, 0 g trans fat, 0 mg cholesterol, 480 mg sodium, 760 mg potassium, 21 g total carbohydrate, 9 g dietary fiber, 8 g sugars, 0 g added sugars, 10 g protein, 240 mg phosphorus

Pan-Toasting Pine Nuts

For extra-nutty taste, toast the pine nuts. The easiest way to do that is to heat a skillet over medium-high heat. No oil is needed. Add the pine nuts and cook while stirring constantly until lightly browned, about 3 minutes. Immediately transfer the toasted pine nuts to a heatproof bowl.

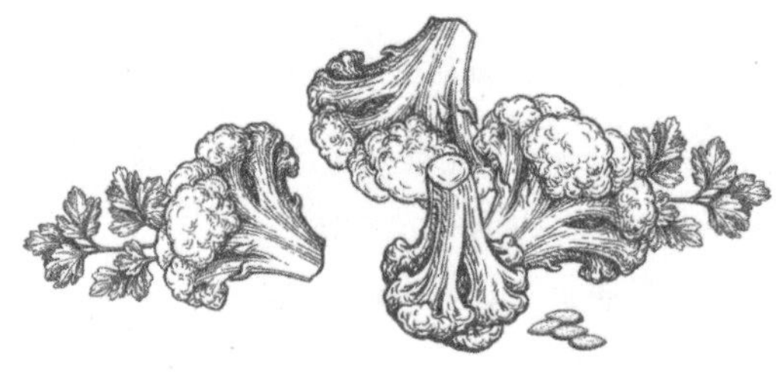

FARMERS' MARKET MUSHROOM FLATBREAD PIZZA

Pizza can fit into a diabetes-friendly eating plan—and a plant-based one. Cheers to that! One of the keys is to load it up with veggies, like mushrooms (even though botanically mushrooms are considered fungi). For this flatbread version, pick up a variety of them, such as baby bellas (crimini mushrooms), shiitake caps, and oyster mushrooms, from your local farmers' market or a natural foods market. (Hint: Using a combination of three types of mushrooms rather than one will provide a more complex and exciting flavor profile.)

SERVES: 4 | SERVING SIZE: 2 slices
PREP TIME: 12 minutes | COOK TIME: 24–26 minutes

- 1½ tablespoons extra-virgin olive oil, divided
- 1 small white onion, very thinly sliced
- 8 ounces sliced fresh mushroom mixture (3 cups)
- ½ teaspoon minced fresh rosemary
- ½ teaspoon sea salt, divided
- 2 (3-ounce) soft whole-grain naan or other whole-grain flatbreads
- ½ cup plant-based ricotta-style cheese*
- 1 large garlic clove, minced
- ¼ cup shredded, plant-based, mozzarella-style cheese*
- 1 teaspoon black sesame seeds
- 8 fresh basil leaves, torn

**Note: Ideally, choose vegan cheese products based on tree nuts.*

DIRECTIONS

1. Heat 1 tablespoon of the oil in a large stick-resistant skillet over medium-high heat. Add the onion and sauté until lightly caramelized, about 5 minutes. Add the mushrooms, rosemary, and ¼ teaspoon of the salt and sauté until the mushrooms are wilted, about 5 minutes. Transfer to a bowl and set aside.
2. Preheat the oven to 450°F. Brush the entire top surface of each flatbread with the remaining ½ tablespoon oil. In a small bowl, stir together the plant-based ricotta-style cheese, garlic, and remaining ¼ teaspoon of the salt. (Hint: If you're following a

sodium-modified eating plan, reduce this added salt to ⅛ teaspoon or less.) Spread mixture onto the flatbreads, leaving about a ¼-inch rim. Top with the plant-based mozzarella-style cheese, mushroom mixture, and sesame seeds.

3. Place both pizzas on a large baking sheet and bake until the cheese is melted and the crust is crisp, about 13–15 minutes. Remove from the oven. Let stand for about 5 minutes to complete the cooking process.
4. Cut each pizza into 4 pieces, sprinkle with the basil, and serve immediately.

NUTRITION INFO
Choices/Exchanges: 2 starch, 1 high fat protein, 1 fat
Per serving: 290 calories, 16 g total fat, 4 g saturated fat, 0 g trans fat, 0 mg cholesterol, 660 mg sodium, 413 mg potassium, 29 g total carbohydrate, 2 g dietary fiber, 4 g sugars, 0 g added sugars, 9 g protein, 157 mg phosphorus

A Citrus Zing

Are you the culinary adventurous type? Try this. When you add the fresh basil to your flatbread pizza, also sprinkle it with freshly grated orange or lemon zest for an aromatic, refreshing, and intriguing citrus zing. If you're not so adventurous, try it anyway!

GRILLED EGGPLANT STEAK

The term "steak" can apply to so many foods now, including these thick, hearty slices of grilled eggplant. They're succulent and fill up the plate even more so than a traditional serving of the beefy version. Savor their Middle Eastern flair paired with a protein-rich appetizer, side, or salad, like hummus, edamame, *Minty Kibbeh-Inspired "Meatballs"* (page 41), or *French Lentil Salad* (page 179). And if you'd like to make this eggplant dish extra luxurious, drizzle it with *Simple Lemony Tahini Sauce* (following recipe).

SERVES: 2 | SERVING SIZE: 2 steaks
PREP TIME: 10 minutes | COOK TIME: 12 to 14 minutes

- 1 large eggplant, cut into 4 thick slices lengthwise (about 6 ounces per slice)
- 1 tablespoon extra-virgin olive oil
- ½ teaspoon freshly ground black pepper, or to taste
- ¼ teaspoon sea salt, or to taste
- ⅛ teaspoon ground cinnamon
- 2 teaspoons pine nuts, pan-toasted
- 1 tablespoon packed small fresh mint leaves
- 2 lemon wedges

DIRECTIONS

1. Prepare an outdoor or indoor grill. Lightly brush the eggplant with the oil using a silicone pastry brush. Sprinkle with the pepper, salt, and cinnamon.
2. Grill over direct medium-high heat until fully cooked through and rich grill marks form, about 6 to 7 minutes per side. Adjust seasoning.
3. Transfer to two plates and sprinkle with the pine nuts and mint. Serve with the lemon wedges on the side.

NUTRITION INFO
Choices/Exchanges: 3 vegetable, 2 fat
Per serving: 170 calories, 9 g total fat, 1 g saturated fat, 0 g trans fat, 0 mg cholesterol, 300 mg sodium, 818 mg potassium, 22 g total carbohydrate, 10 g dietary fiber, 11 g sugars, 0 g added sugars, 4 g protein, 101 mg phosphorus

SIMPLE LEMONY TAHINI SAUCE

- 3 tablespoons tahini
- 2 tablespoons cold water or unsweetened green tea
- 1½ teaspoons lemon juice
- ⅛ teaspoon sea salt

In a small jar, shake together all ingredients. (Makes about ⅓ cup.)

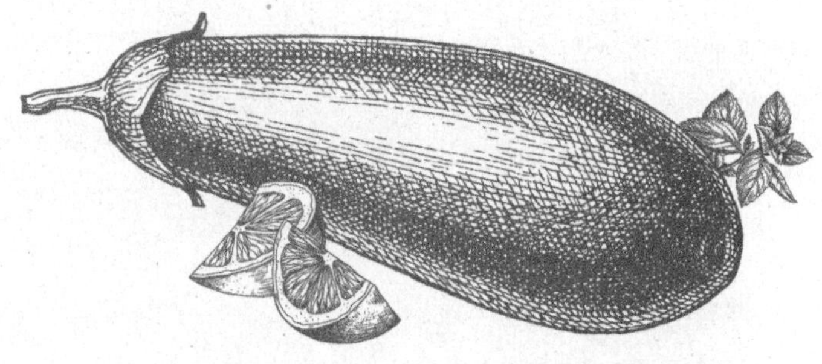

ROASTED VEGETABLE ENCHILADA BAKE

If you're a fan of Mexican-inspired cuisine, you may find yourself moving your hips and singing "La Bamba" about this rather luscious casserole-style dish. The tomatillo salsa gives it delightful tang; the poblano pepper and pinto beans provide rich body; and the spinach and mushrooms impart savoriness and, of course, veggie goodness. The distinctive tastes of cilantro, oregano, and cumin make this recipe unforgettable. If you have room within your personalized plan, take your portion over the top by topping with a dollop of one of my guacamole recipes in this book.

SERVES: 6 | SERVING SIZE: ⅙ of casserole (about 2 cups)
PREP TIME: 18 minutes | COOK TIME: 39 minutes

- 2 teaspoons avocado oil or unrefined peanut oil
- 1 large sweet onion, diced
- 1¼ cups mild or medium tomatillo salsa (salsa verde) of choice, divided
- 12 ounces baby bellas (crimini mushrooms) or white button mushrooms, sliced
- 1 fresh poblano pepper, chopped
- 5 cups packed fresh baby spinach (5 ounces)
- 1 (15-ounce) can reduced-sodium pinto beans, rinsed and drained (1½ cups)
- 3 tablespoons chopped fresh cilantro
- 1 teaspoon finely chopped fresh oregano leaves
- ½ teaspoon ground cumin
- ¼ teaspoon sea salt, or to taste
- 12 (6-inch) corn tortillas
- ½ cup shredded plant-based Monterey Jack or Mexican-style cheese* (2 ounces)

**Note: Ideally, choose vegan cheese products based on tree nuts.*

DIRECTIONS

1. Preheat the oven to 400°F.
2. Heat the oil in a large, deep, stick-resistant skillet over medium-high heat. Add the onion and ¼ cup of the salsa and sauté until the onion is softened, about 8 minutes. Add the mushrooms and poblano pepper and sauté until the mushrooms are softened, about 8 minutes. Stir in the spinach and toss until just wilted, about 1 minute. Add the beans, cilantro, oregano, cumin, and salt, and sauté until fully combined and heated through, about 1 minute. Adjust seasoning.
3. Spread ½ cup of the salsa into a 9- by 13-inch baking dish. Arrange 6 of the tortillas to cover the bottom of the dish. Evenly top with half of the vegetable mixture. Arrange the remaining 6 tortillas on top. Sprinkle with ¼ cup of the salsa. Evenly top with the remaining vegetable mixture. Sprinkle with the cheese. Bake until fully cooked through and the cheese is melted, about 20 minutes. Sprinkle with the remaining ¼ cup of salsa.
4. Cut the casserole into 6 portions and serve.

NUTRITION INFO

Choices/Exchanges: 2 starch, 1 vegetable, 1 fat

Per serving: 240 calories, 5 g total fat, 0 g saturated fat, 0 g trans fat, 0 mg cholesterol, 680 mg sodium, 570 mg potassium, 40 g total carbohydrate, 7 g dietary fiber, 6 g sugars, 0 g added sugars, 8 g protein, 147 mg phosphorus

EGGPLANT AND SPAGHETTI MARINARA

A bowlful of spaghetti can be a carb overload. But there are ways to keep that pasta bowl simple, satisfying, and scrumptious while keeping carbs in check. This recipe offers one of those ways, while turning a typical spaghetti with jarred sauce into something rather special. Garlicky sautéed eggplant is really all it takes to glam up this supper standby and pump up its volume. Using a right-sized amount of spaghetti—and choosing a whole-grain or pulse-based variety—is key to keeping this recipe healthful. And the finish of fresh basil is a delight.

SERVES: 4 | SERVING SIZE: 1¼ cups pasta
PREP TIME: 12 minutes | COOK TIME: 30 minutes

- 1½ cups no-sugar-added marinara sauce of choice
- 1 tablespoon extra-virgin olive oil
- 1 medium (1-pound) eggplant, cut into ½-inch cubes
- 2 garlic cloves, minced
- 1 teaspoon aged balsamic vinegar
- ⅛ teaspoon sea salt, or to taste
- 5 ounces whole-grain or pulse-based spaghetti
- 2 tablespoons thinly sliced fresh basil leaves or 20 small whole fresh basil leaves

DIRECTIONS

1. Bring the marinara sauce to a boil over high heat in a small saucepan. Reduce heat to low, cover, and keep warm.
2. Heat the oil in a large, stick-resistant skillet over medium heat. Add the eggplant, garlic, vinegar, and salt, and sauté until the eggplant is fully softened, about 18 minutes. Adjust seasoning.
3. Meanwhile, in a large saucepan, cook the pasta according to package directions—or "lid-cook" it (page 186). Drain the pasta, reserving ½ cup cooking liquid. Return the pasta to the large dry saucepan and toss with the eggplant mixture, marinara sauce, and desired amount of the reserved cooking liquid. Adjust seasoning.
4. Divide the pasta among four plates or pasta bowls. Sprinkle with the basil and serve.

NUTRITION INFO
Choices/Exchanges: 2½ starch, 1 vegetable, 1 fat
Per serving: 230 calories, 6 g total fat, 1 g saturated fat, 0 g trans fat, 0 mg cholesterol, 470 mg sodium, 450 mg potassium, 40 g total carbohydrate, 8 g dietary fiber, 9 g sugars, 0 g added sugars, 7 g protein, 130 mg phosphorus

Pasta Preparation Tips

Here, I base the nutrition analysis on the use of no added salt to the pasta water while cooking. It can help you keep your sodium intake in better check by leaving it out. However, if you prefer to keep the salt for optimal taste, just keep it in mind when you plan your meals for the day so you stay within a healthful total daily sodium allowance.

For pasta preparation time, stick to the low end of any range given. For example, cook for 9 minutes if the package says to cook for 9–11 minutes. This will mean your pasta will be al dente (just cooked through). That suggests it will have a more enjoyable texture and a lower glycemic index than if you cooked pasta till fully softened. That's helpful when trying to manage a healthy blood glucose level.

CREAMY MEDITERRANEAN RADIATORE

Chickpeas are like magic beans—they act like cream in this pasta dish. And you'll be amazed at the creaminess of it. The dish seems downright decadent without needing a drop of any cream … or butter or cheese. While chickpeas provide the velvetiness of the sauce, baby spinach creates extra interest, color, and nutrient richness. And the Mediterranean accents of fragrant rosemary, zesty lemon, and toasty pine nuts take the flavor of this comforting pasta over the top.

SERVES: 6 I SERVING SIZE: 1 rounded cup
PREP TIME: 16 minutes I COOK TIME: 13 minutes

- 1 (15-ounce) can chickpeas (garbanzo beans), gently
- rinsed and drained, divided (1½ cups)
- 1¼ cups no-sugar-added marinara sauce of choice
- ½ cup low-sodium vegetable broth
- 1 tablespoon lemon juice + zest of 1 lemon
- 1 teaspoon minced fresh rosemary
- 8 ounces dry whole-grain or pulse-based radiatore or rotini pasta
- 5 cups packed fresh baby spinach or finely chopped
- Swiss chard leaves (5 ounces)
- ¼ teaspoon + ⅛ teaspoon sea salt, or to taste
- ¼ teaspoon freshly ground black pepper, or to taste
- 2½ tablespoons pine nuts, pan-toasted

DIRECTIONS

1. Add 1 cup of the chickpeas, the marinara sauce, broth, lemon juice, and rosemary to a blender. Cover and purée until velvety smooth, at least 2 minutes. Pour the creamy marinara sauce into a medium saucepan. Bring to a boil over high heat. Cover, reduce heat to low, and simmer for about 12 minutes.
2. Meanwhile, cook the radiatore in a large saucepan according to package directions–or "lid-cook" it (page 186)–until al dente. Drain the pasta.
3. Return the pasta to the large dry saucepan over medium heat. Add the creamy marinara sauce and the remaining chickpeas and toss to coat. Add the spinach and salt and toss to coat while cooking until the spinach just wilts, about 1½ minutes. Adjust seasoning.

4. Transfer the pasta to a large serving bowl or individual bowls, sprinkle with the pepper, lemon zest, and pine nuts, and serve.

NUTRITION INFO
Choices/Exchanges: 3 starch, 1 fat
Per serving: 250 calories, 5 g total fat, 0 g saturated fat, 0 g trans fat, 0 mg cholesterol, 490 mg sodium, 380 mg potassium, 43 g total carbohydrate, 7 g dietary fiber, 6 g sugars, 0 g added sugars, 11 g protein, 140 mg phosphorus

DIY Simple No-Sugar-Added Marinara Sauce

In a medium saucepan, cook 2 minced garlic cloves in 2 tablespoons extra-virgin olive oil over medium heat for 1 minute. Add 1 (28-ounce) can crushed tomatoes and a few pinches of sea salt; bring just to a boil over high, then reduce heat to medium-low and simmer for 10 minutes. Stir in 2 tablespoons finely chopped fresh basil. That's it. Enjoy it! (Makes 3 cups.)

SPINACH LOVER'S CACIO E PEPE

Cacio e pepe is a popular Roman pasta dish. It basically means "cheese and pepper." The pepper isn't an afterthought; it's a key ingredient. This loose interpretation of the classic includes the addition of baby spinach . . . lots of it! While traditionally you'll find cacio e pepe made with regular bucatini, spaghetti, or tagliolini, here you'll use a fun-shaped pasta for added interest. For a punch of wholesome plant protein, choose red lentil rotini or other pulse-based pasta. The recipe is so simple, yet so tasty.

SERVES: 2 | SERVING SIZE: 1½ cups
PREP TIME: 6 minutes | COOK TIME: 10 minutes

- 8 cups cold water
- 3½ ounces dry whole-wheat or red lentil rotini
- 1 (5-ounce) package fresh baby spinach
- 2 teaspoons extra-virgin olive oil
- 1 teaspoon freshly ground black pepper
- ¼ teaspoon sea salt, or to taste
- ¼ cup grated vegan Parmesan-style cheese or other aged plant-based cheese*
- 2 lemon wedges (optional)

**Note: Ideally, choose vegan cheese products based on tree nuts.*

DIRECTIONS

1. Add the water to a large saucepan. Bring to a boil over high heat. Stir in the rotini and cook according to package directions, about 8 minutes. Drain the pasta using a strainer. Set aside.
2. Add the spinach to the large dry saucepan. Place over medium heat. Cook while stirring until the spinach is slightly wilted, about 1 minute. Add the drained pasta, oil, pepper, and salt, and cook while stirring until the spinach is fully wilted, about 1 minute. Stir in the plant-based cheese.
3. Transfer to a bowl and, if desired, serve with lemon wedges.

NUTRITION INFO
Choices/Exchanges: 2 starch, 2 vegetable, 1 fat
Per serving: 270 calories, 8 g total fat, 2 g saturated fat, 0 g trans fat, 0 mg cholesterol, 430 mg sodium, 541 mg potassium, 45 g total carbohydrate, 7 g dietary fiber, 1 g sugars, 0 g added sugars, 10 g protein, 209 mg phosphorus

Black Pepper Benefits

Even when a recipe doesn't specifically call for black pepper, you can absolutely add it. Besides offering its distinctive kick in the palate, black pepper provides polyphenols, which are antioxidants, and a compound called piperine, which may play a role in diabetes treatment. For the biggest flavor and nutritional benefit, get a pepper mill so you can grind pepper as needed rather than using pre-ground pepper.

Bonus Tip: For additional culinary flair, gently toast whole peppercorns in a dry skillet over medium heat until fragrant, about 2 minutes or so. Then coarsely grind it using a pepper mill or a mortar and pestle. It'll make this recipe extra special.

VEGGIE CHOW FUN

Chow fun is a Cantonese dish based on rice noodles. And you can't beat a bowl of noodles in the wintertime—or anytime, for that matter. This nutrient-packed version is heavy on the veggies, including eggplant, baby bok choy, oyster mushrooms, and scallions, and uses brown rice noodles. The finish of fresh basil and toasted sesame seeds is so inviting. Full of textures and rich flavor, this chow fun really is fun for your taste buds!

SERVES: 4 | SERVING SIZE: 1¼ cups
PREP TIME: 22 minutes | COOK TIME: 20 minutes

- ½ cup low-sodium vegetable broth
- 2 tablespoons naturally brewed soy sauce, or to taste
- 2 tablespoons unsweetened applesauce
- 6 ounces dry flat, short, and wide brown rice noodles or broken pad Thai brown rice noodles
- 2 tablespoons avocado oil or sunflower oil, divided
- 3 cups diced eggplant, unpeeled (8 ounces)
- ⅛ teaspoon sea salt, or to taste
- 2 large garlic cloves, minced
- 2 teaspoons freshly grated gingerroot
- 2 small bunches fresh baby bok choy, thinly sliced (2¾ cups sliced)
- 1 cup oyster mushrooms, separated, or sliced shiitake mushroom caps
- 4 scallions, green and white parts, thinly sliced on the diagonal
- 3 tablespoons thinly sliced fresh basil
- 1½ teaspoons white or black sesame seeds, pan-toasted

DIRECTIONS

1. Whisk together the broth, soy sauce, and applesauce in a liquid measuring cup. Set aside.
2. Prepare the noodles according to package directions. Rinse under cold water (or toss with ice cubes to cool), drain, and transfer to a medium serving bowl. Set aside. (Note: If noodles sit too long and become sticky, rinse and drain again.)
3. Heat 2 teaspoons of the oil in a wok or large skillet over medium-high heat. Add the eggplant and sauté until just cooked through, about 5 minutes. Transfer to a plate. Set aside.

4. Place the wok over high heat and add 2 teaspoons of the oil. Add the noodles and stir-fry for 15 seconds. Add half the reserved sauce and the salt and stir to evenly coat noodles, about 45 seconds. Transfer the noodles back into the serving bowl.
5. Replace the wok over high heat and add the remaining 2 teaspoons oil. Add the garlic and ginger and stir-fry for 30 seconds. Add the bok choy, mushrooms, scallions, and the reserved eggplant and stir-fry until all vegetables are fully cooked, about 2 minutes. Return the noodles to the pan along with the reserved sauce and toss to coat while cooking until fully heated and combined, about 1 minute. Stir in the basil. Adjust seasoning.
6. Transfer to the serving bowl or individual bowls and sprinkle with the sesame seeds. Serve while hot with additional soy sauce on the side, if desired.

NUTRITION INFO

Choices/Exchanges: 2½ starch, 1 vegetable, 1½ fat

Per serving: 270 calories, 9 g total fat, 1 g saturated fat, 0 g trans fat, 0 mg cholesterol, 580 mg sodium, 390 mg potassium, 43 g total carbohydrate, 6 g dietary fiber, 4 g sugars, 0 g added sugars, 7 g protein, 70 mg phosphorus

SPRING GARDEN "RISOTTO" WITH ASPARAGUS

Traditional risotto uses arborio rice, which is a starchy, Italian processed grain. This recipe goes the non-traditional route. Consider it a creamy risotto-inspired entrée. It lets the flavor of nature's best play the lead role, especially the asparagus. Plus, you don't need to stand at the stove and stir continuously as traditional risotto requires. A simplified rice cooking technique is used here. The result: a pleasurable dish full of spring garden deliciousness. Pair it with grilled tofu skewers or *Minty Kibbeh-Inspired "Meatballs"* (page 41) to round out the meal.

SERVES: 6 | SERVING SIZE: 1 cup
PREP TIME: 18 minutes | COOK TIME: 1 hour

- 1 tablespoon extra-virgin olive oil
- 1 medium yellow onion, finely chopped
- 2 teaspoons fresh lemon juice
- 1 teaspoon sea salt, divided
- 1½ cups uncooked short-grain brown rice
- 3½ cups low-sodium vegetable broth, divided
- 1 cup steamed cauliflower floret pieces, warm or at room temperature
- ¼ cup fresh mint leaves + 6 fresh mint sprigs
- ¼ cup fresh basil leaves
- 12 asparagus spears, cut into ½-inch pieces on the diagonal, ends trimmed
- 6 sun-dried tomato halves, extra-thinly sliced, do not rehydrate
- 1 tablespoon vegan butter
- 2 tablespoons grated vegan Parmesan-style cheese or other aged plant-based cheese*

**Note: Ideally, choose vegan cheese products based on tree nuts.*

DIRECTIONS

1. Heat the oil in a large saucepan over medium heat. Add the onion, lemon juice, and ¼ teaspoon of the salt and sauté until the onion is softened, about 8 minutes. Stir in the

rice, 3 cups of the broth, and the remaining ¾ teaspoon salt, increase heat to high, and bring to a boil. Cover, reduce heat to low, and simmer for 30 minutes. The rice will not be fully cooked.

2. Meanwhile, add the steamed cauliflower, mint leaves, basil, and the remaining ½ cup broth to a blender. Cover and purée until smooth.
3. Stir the cauliflower-herb purée, asparagus, and sundried tomatoes into the rice mixture, cover, and simmer over low heat until the rice is cooked through yet still slightly chewy, about 20 minutes more. Stir in the vegan butter and cheese. Adjust seasoning.
4. Spoon onto individual plates or bowls, top with the mint sprigs, and serve.

NUTRITION INFO

Choices/Exchanges: 2 starch, 1½ vegetable, 1 fat

Per serving: 260 calories, 6 g total fat, 2 g saturated fat, 0 g trans fat, 0 mg cholesterol, 510 mg sodium, 334 mg potassium, 45 g total carbohydrate, 5 g dietary fiber, 4 g sugars, 0 g added sugars, 6 g protein, 193 mg phosphorus

VEGETABLE MOUSSE "MEATLOAF"

A classic American comfort food is meatloaf. But what's a plant-based eater supposed to have? That's easy, *Vegetable Mousse "Meatloaf."* I started making it from leftover non-starchy veggie scraps that needed to be used quickly. But I enjoyed it so much that I crafted the concept into a "real" recipe to use anytime. These loaves are moist and mousse-like on the inside and lovable as is or with bonus toppings. Don't expect them to taste like the meaty kind, but do expect the results to be vegan comfort food worthy of becoming a go-to main dish.

SERVES: 4 I SERVING SIZE: 1 personal-sized loaf
PREP TIME: 15 minutes I COOK TIME: 50 minutes

- 1 medium (8-ounce) zucchini, sliced
- 2 cups packed, small cauliflower florets (6 ounces)
- 8 ounces baby bellas (crimini mushrooms), halved or sliced
- 1½ ounces fresh chard or spinach leaves without stems, torn (2 cups packed torn)
- 2 scallions, green and white parts, sliced
- ⅓ cup chickpea (garbanzo bean) flour
- 3 tablespoons chia seeds
- 2 garlic cloves, minced
- ¾ teaspoon + ⅛ teaspoon sea salt, or to taste
- ½ teaspoon freshly ground black pepper
- 2 tablespoons extra-virgin olive oil

DIRECTIONS

1. Preheat the oven to 425°F. Line a baking sheet with a silicone baking mat or unbleached parchment paper.
2. Add the zucchini and cauliflower to a food processor. Cover and pulse several times until finely chopped. Add the remaining ingredients and blend until well combined and mixture resembles a well-textured pesto. Note: If you're following a sodium-modified eating plan, use just ¾ teaspoon or less sea salt.

3. On the baking sheet, form the mixture into 4 well-rounded loaves, about ⅞ cup each. (Hint: Measure the ⅞-cup mixture into a 1-cup dry measure and tap out onto the baking sheet into four 3¾-inch diameter loaves. Alternatively, form into 8 mini-loaves.)
4. Roast until cooked through and browned, about 50 minutes (or 40 minutes for mini-loaves). Remove from the oven and let stand at least 5 minutes to complete the cooking process.
5. Gently transfer the loaves to a serving platter. Serve as is or with toppings.

NUTRITION INFO
Choices/Exchanges: 3 vegetable, 2 fat
Per serving: 170 calories, 11 g total fat, 1.5 g saturated fat, 0 g trans fat, 0 mg cholesterol, 550 mg sodium, 715 mg potassium, 14 g total carbohydrate, 5 g dietary fiber, 4 g sugars, 0 g added sugars, 6 g protein, 192 mg phosphorus

Mod "Meatloaf" Toppings

For an extra punch of pizzaz on the plate and your palate, pair your vegetable loaves with toppings as you wish. Try these pleasing combos or one of your own:

- Plant-based sour cream + fresh chives and/or sautéed minced chard stems
- Naturally brewed soy sauce with a splash of rice vinegar + scallions
- *Simple Lemony Tahini Sauce* (page 104) + pomegranate arils + fresh mint leaves
- Dairy-free pesto sauce + extra-thinly sliced grape tomatoes or sun-dried tomato bits
- Chimichurri sauce + extra-thinly sliced red hot chili peppers

BLACKENED ORANGE AND GINGER TOFU FILETS

If you're looking for a plant protein-packed entrée that can be a stand-in for chicken, fish, or turkey, these sassy tofu filets are dinnertime dazzlers. The orange and ginger are flavor highlights. But the charry appearance makes them crave-worthy. Plan to make these plant-based filets at your next cookout—or cook-in. They're delightful paired with grilled asparagus or *Spring Asparagus Stir-Fry* (page 225) and a whole grain, like brown basmati rice. Plus, they can be cooked in advance, chilled, sliced, and served on top of a lunchtime salad bowl. (Hint: Enjoy two filets for a power-packed meal!)

SERVES: 4 | SERVING SIZE: 1 filet
PREP TIME: 12 minutes | COOK TIME: 12 minutes

- 1 (14-ounce) package extra-firm organic tofu,* squeezed well of any excess liquid
- 1 tablespoon toasted sesame oil
- ½ teaspoon sea salt, divided
- 2 tablespoons freshly squeezed orange or mandarin orange juice with pulp or pear nectar
- ½ teaspoon grated orange or mandarin orange zest
- 1 teaspoon freshly grated gingerroot
- ¼ teaspoon freshly ground black pepper, divided
- 1 scallion, white part minced, green part extra-thinly sliced, separated
- ½ small red hot chili pepper, extra-thinly sliced

**Note: Use tofu that's made from soybeans (traditional), chickpeas, or pumpkin seeds.*

DIRECTIONS

1. Preheat a grill or grill pan over medium-high heat. Cut the tofu block into 4 filets (first cut the block like it's a burger bun, then halve it). Brush with the sesame oil and sprinkle with ¼ teaspoon + ⅛ teaspoon of the salt.
2. In a small bowl, stir together the orange juice and zest, ginger, black pepper, white part of the scallions, and the remaining ⅛ teaspoon salt.

3. Grill the tofu filets until rich grill marks form on the bottom side, about 5 minutes. Flip over; spread (using a long-handled spoon) with all of the orange-ginger sauce; and grill until rich grill marks form on this flip side, about 5 minutes total. Flip over and grill until the orange-ginger side is well caramelized (blackened), about 2 minutes.
4. Transfer the grilled tofu filets onto a platter, sprinkle with the green part of the scallion and chili pepper, and serve.

NUTRITION INFO
Choices/Exchanges: 1½ very lean protein, 2 fat
Per serving: 140 calories, 9 g total fat, 1 g saturated fat, 0 g trans fat, 0 mg cholesterol, 300 mg sodium, 47 mg potassium, 4 g total carbohydrate, 2 g dietary fiber, 1 g sugars, 0 g added sugars, 10 g protein, 6 mg phosphorus

What is Orange Zest?

Orange zest is the vibrant, grated, brightly-colored outer layer of the orange peel that's full of citrusy aroma, essential oils, and concentrated, tangy orange favor with a hint of bitterness, It has potential anti-inflammatory and antioxidant benefits, too.

After washing and patting dry an orange, grate it using a zester, grater, or peeler—and don't use any of the white pithy part under the outer orange layer. It's intensely flavored so you don't need much of it. Use it as an aromatic flavoring ingredient in savory recipes, like pilafs and marinades, or sweet dishes, like muffins and cakes. It's delicious in chocolaty baked goodies, FYI!

Tip: Whenever you'rejuicing an orange, grate the peel first. You'll be surprised at all of the ways you can use the zest. If you can't use it right away, freeze it for later.

BARBECUED BONELESS TEMPEH RIBS

If you've nixed barbecued ribs out of your healthful eating plan, now you can plop them back in. These ribs are still barbecue-y and finger-licking. But they're boneless, 100 percent plant-based, and super easy to make. Just slice the tempeh, brush with BBQ sauce, marinate for 1 hour, and grill. Even true rib fanatics will be pleasantly surprised by the texture and appearance of these bites—no bones about it. Serve these alongside appealing veggie sides, like *Tricolor Coleslaw* (page 197) or *Grape Tomato Succotash* (page 231).

SERVES: 2 | SERVING SIZE: 6 ribs
PREP TIME: 4 minutes (+ 1 hour marinating time) | COOK TIME: 14 to 15 minutes

- 1 (8-ounce) package tempeh, cut crosswise into 12 slices
- ¼ cup no-sugar-added barbecue sauce or *Fruit-Sweetened BBQ Sauce* (page 58), divided
- ⅛ teaspoon sea salt
- 2 teaspoons minced fresh chives (optional)

DIRECTIONS

1. Lightly brush all surfaces of the tempeh slices with 2 tablespoons of the barbecue sauce. Sprinkle with the salt. Place into a sealed glass container in the refrigerator to marinate for 1 hour.
2. Preheat a grill or grill-pan over medium heat. On a cut surface of the tempeh ribs, grill until browned, about 8 minutes; flip over, brush with 1 tablespoon barbecue sauce, and grill until browned, about 5 to 6 minutes; flip over again, brush with the remaining 1 tablespoon barbecue sauce, and cook 1 minute more.
3. Pile up the ribs in the center of a serving bowl, sprinkle with the chives, if desired, and serve.

NUTRITION INFO

Choices/Exchanges: 1 carbohydrate, 3 very lean protein, ½ fat

Per serving: 200 calories, 6 g total fat, 1.5 g saturated fat, 0 g trans fat, 0 mg cholesterol, 450 mg sodium, 403 mg potassium, 19 g total carbohydrate, 9 g dietary fiber, 0 g sugars, 0 g added sugars, 22 g protein, 302 mg phosphorus

Saucy Swaps

These tempeh ribs work well with so many other sauces. Go ahead and try your favorites, or one of these: plant-based pesto, marinara, chimichurri, mole, or stir-fry sauce. Prepare it just like in this recipe. Have fun with it.

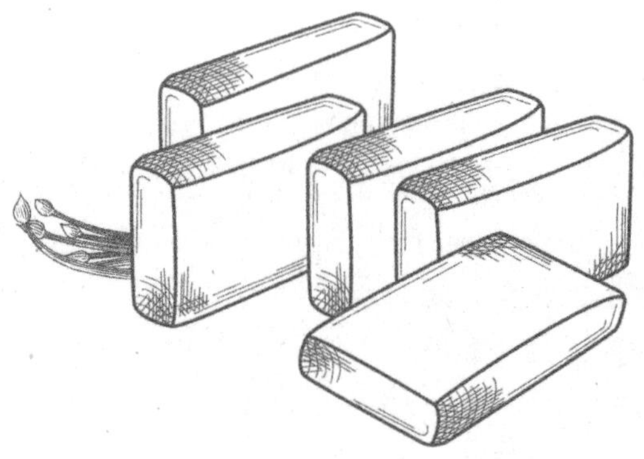

Main Dishes: Burgers, Sandwiches, and Wraps

BIG VEGAN BURGER SLIDERS

No wimpy patties here. The big slider patties are based on black beans, offering lots of filling satisfaction thanks to the duo of fiber and protein. Chia seeds and chickpea flour provide body, while onion, garlic, coriander, and smoked paprika kick up the scrumptiousness. Open wide and serve the sliders with whatever toppings you enjoy, like *Special Sauce* (following recipe), vine-ripened tomato slices, and fresh baby arugula. And if you're into cheesiness, there's no "rule" that says you can't go "off recipe" and add a bit more vegan cheese to your serving. Pair your slider with non-starchy grilled veggies or a leafy side salad to make it a meal.

SERVES: 4 | SERVING SIZE: 1 slider
PREP TIME: 17 minutes | COOK TIME: 17 minutes

- 2 tablespoons sunflower or avocado oil, divided
- 1 small or ½ medium red onion, finely diced
- ½ teaspoon sea salt, divided
- 2 large garlic cloves, minced
- ¾ teaspoon ground coriander
- ¼ teaspoon smoked paprika
- 1 (15-ounce) can no-salt-added black beans, drained

- 2 slices vegan cheese of choice,* divided
- 2 tablespoons fruit-sweetened or no-sugar-added ketchup
- 2 tablespoons chickpea (garbanzo bean) or other flour
- 1½ tablespoons chia seeds
- 4 whole-grain slider rolls, split

**Note: Ideally, choose vegan cheese products based on tree nuts.*

DIRECTIONS

1. Heat 1 tablespoon of the oil in a large cast-iron or other stick-resistant skillet over medium heat. Add the onion and ¼ teaspoon of the salt and cook while stirring until the onion is softened, about 5 minutes. Add the garlic, coriander, and paprika and cook while stirring until fragrant, about 1 minute. Set aside until cool enough to handle.
2. In a large bowl, roughly smash the beans using a potato masher or large fork. Finely dice 1 of the vegan cheese slices and stir into the smashed beans. Add the ketchup, chickpea flour, chia seeds, remaining ¼ teaspoon salt, and the onion mixture, and stir to evenly combine.
3. Form the bean mixture into 4 balls, about ⅓ cup each. On a silicone baking mat-lined pan, or unbleached parchment paper-lined baking pan, press the balls into patties, about 3-inch diameter each. (Hint: You can form the patties in advance, chill for up to 3 days, and then pan-cook when ready.)
4. Heat the remaining 1 tablespoon oil in a large skillet over medium heat. Add the patties and cook until extra-well browned and crisped, about 4½ to 5 minutes per side, adding ¼ slice of remaining vegan cheese to each patty after flipping. Serve a cheesy patty in each roll with desired toppings on the side.

NUTRITION INFO

Choices/Exchanges: 3 starch, 2 fat

Per serving: 310 calories, 14 g total fat, 2.5 g saturated fat, 0 g trans fat, 0 mg cholesterol, 595 mg sodium, 459 mg potassium, 43 g total carbohydrate, 7 g dietary fiber, 5 g sugars, 0 g added sugars, 11 g protein, 132 mg phosphorus

SPECIAL SAUCE

- ¼ cup fruit-sweetened or no-sugar-added ketchup
- ¼ cup vegan mayo or aquafaba "mayo"
- 2 tablespoons Dijon mustard

Stir together the ketchup, mayo, and mustard and chill in the refrigerator in a sealed container or jar until ready to serve. (Makes about ⅔ cup.)

ALL-AMERICAN PORTABELLA CHEESEBURGERS

Okay, so these are not technically cheeseburgers. But if you're eating plant-based, they're a tasty way to sink your teeth into 100 percent burger-style satisfaction at your next cookout (or cook-in!). The "meatiness" comes from grilled portabella mushroom caps, which will please both vegetarians and nonvegetarians. Go ahead and mix-n-match toppings as you like, too. For instance, instead of salad greens, try microgreens. In lieu of ketchup, spread with guacamole. And for extra smokiness, grill the buns, not just the portabellas.

SERVES: 4 | SERVING SIZE: 1 "cheeseburger"
PREP TIME: 10 minutes | COOK TIME: 8 minutes

- 4 large (5-inch) portabella mushrooms, stems removed
- 1 tablespoon extra-virgin olive oil
- 4 thin slices vegan cheddar-style cheese*
- 4 sprouted whole-grain or whole-wheat hamburger buns, split
- ½ medium red onion, thinly sliced
- 2 cups packed fresh spring mix or other salad greens
- ¼ cup fruit-sweetened or no-sugar-added ketchup

**Note: Ideally, choose vegan cheese products based on tree nuts.*

DIRECTIONS

1. Preheat a grill or grill pan over medium-high heat. (Hint: If using a grill pan, grill in batches.)
2. Rub the rounded side of mushrooms with the oil. Do not remove mushroom gills.
3. Grill the mushrooms, rounded side down, until grill marks form, about 4 minutes. Flip over the mushrooms, top with the cheese, and grill until softened, about 4 minutes. If desired, transfer cooked mushrooms to a cooling rack (that's placed on a rimmed baking sheet) to allow excess liquids to drip off for 2 minutes.
4. Place cheesy portabellas on the bottom bun portions. Top each with the sliced onion, ½ cup salad greens, and the bun tops. Or stuff the buns in any order you prefer. Serve with the ketchup on the side— or consider pairing with *Special Sauce* (page 124).

NUTRITION INFO

Choices/Exchanges: 2 starch, 1 medium fat protein, ½ fat

Per serving: 260 calories, 11 g total fat, 1.5 g saturated fat, 0 g trans fat, 0 mg cholesterol, 480 mg sodium, 437 mg potassium, 31 g total carbohydrate, 7 g dietary fiber, 6 g sugars, 0 g added sugars, 13 g protein, 193 mg phosphorus

The "Sunshine" Vitamin

You'll appreciate knowing that portabella mushrooms provide vitamin D—"the sunshine vitamin." In fact, they're one of the only natural sources of the vitamin found in the produce section! When exposed to UV light by growers, it enhances their amount of vitamin D. Why is this important? Vitamin D may play a beneficial role in overcoming insulin resistance. That's especially helpful when your body isn't getting its daily dose of the vitamin naturally from the sun.

BÁNH MÌ-STYLE, PLANT-BASED HOT DOGS

If you haven't tried a plant-based hot dog in a while (or ever!), here's your chance. There are now many options available that frankly taste like smoky franks. Ideally, choose a regular- instead of jumbo-sized version. Of course, you can serve a plant-based dawg in your favorite all-American style; but you'll be truly delighted by this Vietnamese version. It's a twist on a traditional *bánh mì*, which is a crusty sandwich usually served with sliced pork. The spicy vegan mayo and fresh cilantro finish here makes these hot dogs aromatic and inviting.

SERVES: 4 | SERVING SIZE: 1 topped hot dog
PREP TIME: 14 minutes | COOK TIME: about 6 minutes

- 3 tablespoons vegan mayo or aquafaba "mayo"
- 2 teaspoons natural hot chili sauce or harissa sauce, or to taste
- 4 (4½-inch) whole-grain French baguette portions or hot dog buns, split partway open
- ½ cup packed (0.5 ounces) fresh mizuna, tatsoi, or baby arugula
- 1 (4½-inch) portion English cucumber, cut into long skinny strips
- ¼ cup shredded carrots
- 4 (1.5-ounce) non-GMO plant-based hot dogs
- ¼ cup fresh cilantro leaves or small sprigs
- 4 lime wedges

DIRECTIONS

1. In a small bowl, stir together the vegan mayo and hot chili sauce.
2. Thinly spread half of the spicy mayo into the baguettes. Stuff with the leafy salad greens, cucumber, and carrots.
3. Prepare the plant-based hot dogs according to package directions.
4. Stuff the hot dogs into the baguettes, drizzle with the remaining spicy mayo mixture, and top with the cilantro. Serve with the lime wedges on the side.

NUTRITION INFO

Choices/Exchanges: 1½ starch, 1 vegetable, 1 lean protein, 2 fat

Per serving: 290 calories, 15 g total fat, 2 g saturated fat, 0 g trans fat, 0 mg cholesterol, 470 mg sodium, 120 mg potassium, 25 g total carbohydrate, 2 g dietary fiber, 4 g sugars, 0 g added sugars, 9 g protein, 156 mg phosphorus

Too Much Dough?

For this recipe, just pinch out some of the bready insides of the baguettes, creating four baguette "shells," about 1.5 ounces each. Reserve the soft bread pieces for other use, such as toasted bread cubes/croutons for a salad. You can do this same thing for nearly any recipe calling for a baguette, boule, other whole bread loaves, or buns.

Want to make croutons? Simply toss the bread pieces with a drizzling of extra-virgin olive oil, plus Italian seasoning, garlic powder, and a pinch of sea salt, to taste; and bake in a 375°F oven until golden brown, about 18 minutes.

STUFFED VEGGIE AND HUMMUS SANDWICH

Non-starchy vegetables can transform an ordinary sandwich into an extraordinary one . . . even an overstuffed one! And don't worry, if you find it too challenging to eat this overstuffed sandwich, simply serve some tomato and cucumber on the side instead. Beyond the generous veggie helping, there's another ingredient that may surprise you here: raw shelled hemp seeds (also called hemp hearts). They're low in carbs and provide heart-healthy fats, and when stirred into the hummus, they give the sandwich an extra punch of protein.

SERVES: 1 | SERVING SIZE: 1 sandwich
PREP TIME: 10 minutes | COOK TIME: 0 minutes

- ¼ cup hummus of choice (see recipes in this book)
- 1 tablespoon raw shelled hemp seeds or sesame seeds
- 2 thin slices sprouted whole-grain or whole-wheat bread
- 1 large, thin red onion slice, separated into rings
- 1 plum tomato, thinly sliced
- 1 (3-inch) piece English cucumber, unpeeled, thinly sliced into coins
- Pinch of sea salt
- Pinch of sumac (a Middle Eastern spice) or paprika

DIRECTIONS

1. In a small bowl, stir together the hummus and hemp seeds.
2. Spread the hummus mixture onto both bread slices. Top one bread slice with the onion, tomato, and cucumber. Sprinkle with the salt and sumac. Top with the other bread slice, hummus side down.
3. Serve whole or sliced diagonally in half.

NUTRITION INFO

Choices/Exchanges: 3 starch, 2 medium fat protein, 1 fat

Per serving: 350 calories, 15 g total fat, 1.5 g saturated fat, 0 g trans fat, 0 mg cholesterol, 560 mg sodium, 789 mg potassium, 47 g total carbohydrate, 8 g dietary fiber, 5 g sugars, 0 g added sugars, 17 g protein, 318 mg phosphorus

Which Hummus to Buy

If you choose to purchase hummus rather than prepare homemade hummus, just keep it real! If you see ingredients that your body doesn't need, like the preservative potassium sorbate or the thickener guar gum, ideally pick a different brand.

JALAPEÑO-PEANUT HUMMUS WITH FRESH HERBS

- 1 (15-ounce) can no-salt-added chickpeas (garbanzo beans), drained
- 1 small jalapeño pepper, with or without seeds
- 1 large garlic clove, chopped
- 1 to 2 tablespoons creamy, natural, no-sugar-added peanut butter
- Juice of 1 small lemon (2 tablespoons)
- ¼ cup cold water or unsweetened green tea
- ½ teaspoon sea salt, or to taste
- 3 tablespoons chopped fresh cilantro or flat-leaf parsley

Add all of the ingredients except the cilantro to a food processor or blender. Cover, purée until velvety smooth, at least 2 minutes, adding more water by the tablespoonful only if necessary. Transfer to a serving bowl, sprinkle with the cilantro, and serve. (Makes 6 servings, ¼ cup each, when eaten as a dip.)

NUTRITION INFO

Choices/Exchanges: ½ starch, ½ vegetable, ½ fat

Per serving: 80 calories, 2.5 g total fat, 0 g saturated fat, 0 g trans fat, 0 mg cholesterol, 180 mg sodium, 175 mg potassium, 11 g total carbohydrate, 3 g dietary fiber, 0 g sugars, 0 g added sugars, 4 g protein, 65 mg phosphorus

PAN-GRILLED VEGGIE CIABATTA WITH BALSAMIC TOFUNNAISE

Close your eyes and imagine what your perfect plant-based sandwich looks, smells, and tastes like. Now open your eyes. You're looking at the recipe for it! Not only are the colorful grilled vegetables a joy, the tofu-based "mayo" in this sandwich is, too. The *tofunnaise* is creamy like mayo but bursting with flavor from the balsamic vinegar, garlic, and basil. (Hint: You'll want to make this for other sandwiches.) It's a surprisingly delicious complement here to the veggies and avocado.

SERVES: 4 | SERVING SIZE: 1 sandwich
PREP TIME: 18 minutes | COOK TIME: 8 minutes

BALSAMIC TOFUNNAISE

- 4 ounces organic silken tofu, drained (½ cup)
- 2 tablespoons aged balsamic vinegar
- 1 large clove garlic
- 8 large fresh basil leaves

CIABATTA SANDWICH

- 1 medium zucchini, sliced lengthwise into 4 slices
- 1 medium red or yellow bell pepper, cut into 8 pieces
- Organic oil cooking spray
- 1 (10-ounce) unsliced loaf whole-grain ciabatta or whole-wheat Italian baguette, split
- 1 Hass avocado, peeled, pitted, and sliced
- ¼ teaspoon sea salt
- ¼ cup thinly sliced red onion

DIRECTIONS

1. To make the tofunnaise, purée the tofu, vinegar, garlic, and basil in a blender until smooth. Refrigerate the balsamic tofunnaise until ready to use.

2. Heat a grill pan or outdoor grill over medium-high heat. Spritz the zucchini and bell pepper pieces with cooking spray (or extra-lightly brush with extra-virgin olive oil). Grill the vegetables until cooked through and lightly charred, about 4 minutes per side. Set aside.
3. Pinch out 2 ounces of the fluffy dough from inside of the ciabatta to create 8 ounces of bread for use in this recipe. (Reserve the 2 ounces of doughy bread pieces for another purpose, such as making bread crumbs.)
4. Spread the tofunnaise evenly on both cut surfaces of the bread. Top the bottom bread portion with the zucchini, peppers, avocado, salt, and onion. Place the other bread portion on top and skewer with long toothpicks or small bamboo skewers to secure. Cut into 4 pieces and serve.

NUTRITION INFO

Choices/Exchanges: 2 starch, 1 vegetable, 1 medium fat protein

Per serving: 250 calories, 9 g total fat, 1.5 g saturated fat, 0 g trans fat, 0 mg cholesterol, 370 mg sodium, 570 mg potassium, 34 g total carbohydrate, 8 g dietary fiber, 8 g sugars, 0 g added sugars, 11 g protein, 195 mg phosphorus

Make Ahead

You can prepare the tofunnaise (Step 1) and grill the vegetables (Step 2) in advance. Keep both in sealed jars or containers in the refrigerator for up to 3 days. And if you do decide to make these in advance, consider doubling them so you can enjoy them in other meals.

SLOPPY SAUTÉED EGGPLANT AND PEPPER SANDWICH

This sandwich is intentionally sloppy. Think Sloppy Joe, but better! The recipe is actually a nontraditional twist on a Philly cheesesteak sandwich, though it's messier and overloaded with delicious veggies instead of beef. The sloppiness of it all makes it seem decadent. To top that off, there's just enough plant-based cheesiness and creaminess to add desirable comfort. Though feel free to go for extra cheesiness, if you prefer; just choose a plant-based cheese option that's based on nuts rather than coconut. Grab a couple napkins!

SERVES: 4 | SERVING SIZE: 1 sandwich
PREP TIME: 15 minutes | COOK TIME: 23 minutes

- 4 (2-ounce) whole-wheat or other whole-grain sandwich rolls, split
- 1 ounce plant-based provolone- or mozzarella-style cheese, sliced or shredded* (¼ cup shredded)
- 1 tablespoon avocado oil or sunflower oil
- 1 large (1¼-pound) eggplant, unpeeled, cut into 2-inch by ½-inch batons
- 2 large green bell peppers or mixture of green and red bell peppers, thinly sliced
- 1 medium yellow onion, halved, thinly sliced
- ¾ teaspoon freshly ground black pepper, to taste
- 1 tablespoon white balsamic or white wine vinegar, divided
- ¼ teaspoon sea salt, to taste
- 1 recipe *Spicy Sandwich Spread* (following recipe) or ¼ cup plant-based condiment of choice

**Note: Ideally, choose vegan cheese products based on tree nuts.*

DIRECTIONS

1. Toast or pan-grill the rolls. Immediately top with the cheese. Set aside.
2. Heat the oil in a stick-resistant Dutch oven or large deep skillet over medium-high heat. Add the eggplant, bell peppers, onion, black pepper, 2 teaspoons of the vinegar, and the salt. Cover, and cook, stirring twice, until the vegetables are slightly softened, about 12

minutes. Uncover and sauté until the vegetables are fully softened, about 5 minutes. Stir in the remaining 1 teaspoon vinegar while scraping up the browned bits in the pan for 1 minute. Adjust seasoning. (Makes about 4 cups.)

3. Smear each bun with the sandwich spread, fill with the vegetables, and enjoy immediately.

NUTRITION INFO
Choices/Exchanges: 2 starch, 2 vegetable, 1½ fat
Per serving: 270 calories, 8 g total fat, 2.5 g saturated fat, 0 g trans fat, 0 mg cholesterol, 520 mg sodium, 652 mg potassium, 45 g total carbohydrate, 10 g dietary fiber, 11 g sugars, 0 g added sugars, 10 g protein, 58 mg phosphorus

SPICY SANDWICH SPREAD

- 2 tablespoons plain, unsweetened, plant-based Greek-style yogurt
- 1½ teaspoons vegan mayo or aquafaba "mayo"
- 1 small serrano pepper, without seeds, minced
- 1 large garlic clove, minced
- 1 teaspoon white balsamic or white wine vinegar
- ⅛ teaspoon sea salt, to taste

Stir together the plant-based yogurt, vegan mayo, serrano pepper, garlic, vinegar, and salt in a small bowl until well combined. Use as the condiment in *Sloppy Sautéed Eggplant and Pepper Sandwich* and other sandwiches. (Makes 4 servings, 1 tablespoon each.)

NUTRITION INFO
Choices/Exchanges = 0
Per serving: 10 calories, 0.5 g total fat, 0 g saturated fat, 0 g trans fat, 0 mg cholesterol, 90 mg sodium, 15 mg potassium, 1 g total carbohydrate, 0 g dietary fiber, 0 g sugars, 0 g added sugars, 1 g protein, 2 mg phosphorus

CREAMY TARRAGON "CHICKEN" SALAD ON RYE

This "chicken" salad is based on tofu. And since tofu is rather chameleon-like, it provides the ideal plant-protein base for this intriguing take on a chicken salad sandwich. A key here is that you'll combine the tofu with a dressing bursting with flavor, featuring fresh tarragon and nutritional yeast flakes. Another key is to make this in advance. By allowing the flavors to mingle for a day or two in the fridge, this recipe becomes extra lovable.

SERVES: 6 | SERVING SIZE: 1 sandwich
PREP TIME: 15 minutes | COOK TIME: 3 minutes (for pan-toasting almonds)

CREAMY TARRAGON DRESSING

- 3 tablespoons vegan mayo or aquafaba "mayo"
- 3 tablespoons plain, unsweetened plant-based yogurt
- 1½ tablespoons minced fresh tarragon
- 2 teaspoons nutritional yeast flakes
- 2 teaspoons tarragon vinegar or white wine vinegar
- 1½ teaspoons yellow mustard
- ¾ teaspoon sea salt, or to taste
- ½ teaspoon garlic powder
- ½ teaspoon freshly ground black pepper

"CHICKEN" SALAD

- 1 (14-ounce) package firm organic tofu,* drained and squeezed of excess liquid, diced
- 1 medium stalk celery, extra-thinly sliced on the diagonal (½ cup sliced)
- ¼ cup minced Vidalia or other sweet onion
- ⅓ cup sliced natural almonds, pan-toasted
- 12 (1-ounce) thin slices whole-grain rye bread

**Note: Use tofu that's made from soybeans (traditional), chickpeas, or pumpkin seeds.*

DIRECTIONS

1. In a large bowl, stir together all of the *Creamy Tarragon Dressing* ingredients. Note: If you're following a sodium-modified eating plan, use just ½ teaspoon sea salt or less.
2. Add the tofu, celery, and onion, and stir to combine. Chill in the refrigerator until ready to serve. Adjust seasoning.
3. Stir in the almonds. Serve about ½ cup "chicken" salad in each sandwich, using two slices of bread per sandwich. Slice each sandwich in half diagonally and serve.

NUTRITION INFO

Choices/Exchanges: 2 starch 1 medium fat protein, 1 fat

Per serving: 270 calories, 10 g total fat, 1 g saturated fat, 0 g trans fat, 0 mg cholesterol, 695 mg sodium, 191 mg potassium, 33 g total carbohydrate, 2 g dietary fiber, 3 g sugars, 0 g added sugars, 13 g protein, 102 mg phosphorus

Types of Tofu

Tofu is traditionally a soybean curd. However, as the number of plant-based eaters has grown, so too have the varieties of tofu available. Some are based on other main ingredients instead of soybeans, such as pumpkin seeds (hello, Pumfu!) and chickpeas. Many flavor-infused fresh and baked, ready-to-eat versions exist now too, such as spiced Moroccan and tangy teriyaki flavors. It's an exciting time for tofu!

SWEET POTATO TORTILLA SPIRALS WITH BELL PEPPER AVOCADO-"CRÈME" SAUCE

Years ago, after eating at a tiny Mexican restaurant in the West Village of New York City, I was inspired to create this recipe to mimic the meal where I totally wanted to lick my plate clean in public! More eye-appealing than any ordinary burrito, this delicious translation is like art on the plate—and the palate. The sunset-hued sauce that goes with it is not just gorgeous, it's bursting with antioxidants and versatility. Be sure to whirl up the dreamy sauce (follow Step 3) to pair with other recipes, too.

SERVES: 6 | SERVING SIZE: 2 spirals
PREP TIME: 20 minutes | COOK TIME: 7 to 9 minutes

- 1⅓ cups canned vegetarian refried beans
- 3 large (10-inch) whole-wheat or other whole-grain flour tortillas
- 1½ cups diced cooked sweet potato with skin, warm or cool
- 1 Hass avocado, peeled, pitted, and thinly sliced, divided
- 4 scallions, thinly sliced, green and white parts divided
- 2 cups finely shredded romaine lettuce
- ¼ cup chopped fresh cilantro
- 1½ teaspoons peanut or avocado oil
- 1 large red bell pepper, chopped
- 1 small jalapeño pepper with seeds, sliced
- Juice of 1 lime (about 2 tablespoons)
- ⅛ teaspoon sea salt (optional)

DIRECTIONS

1. Spread the beans over the entire surface of each tortilla. (Heating the refried beans is not required.) Then, again over the entire surface, add the sweet potato, half of the avocado, the green part of the scallions, lettuce, and cilantro.
2. As tightly as possible, roll each filled tortilla without folding in sides. Slice diagonally with a bread knife into 4 pieces each. Set aside.
3. Heat the oil in a medium stick-resistant skillet over medium-high heat. Add the bell pepper, jalapeño, white part of the scallions, lime juice, and, if using, salt, and sauté until the peppers are softened, about 6–8 minutes. Transfer the pepper mixture (including

any browned bits) and the remaining avocado half into a blender. Pulse until combined, then purée for 1 minute on high speed. If necessary, add up to 2 tablespoons cold water for proper blending.

4. Spoon the warm (or room temperature) bell pepper avocado-"crème" sauce onto each of 6 plates. Arrange 2 burrito spirals, cut side down, on each sauce portion, and serve at room temperature. Leftovers taste great!

NUTRITION INFO
Choices/Exchanges: 2 starch, 1 vegetable, 1 fat
Per serving: 240 calories, 8 g total fat, 1.5 g saturated fat, 0 g trans fat, 0 mg cholesterol, 590 mg sodium, 550 mg potassium, 35 g total carbohydrate, 10 g dietary fiber, 4 g sugars, 0 g added sugars, 7 g protein, 105 mg phosphorus

Quick Tips

Boil the sweet potato in advance so it's recipe ready. Or, if you haven't done so, just zap a large sweet potato in the microwave. You also can make the burrito spirals up to 2 days in advance. Wrap each tightly and chill. (Hint: They actually slice better when chilled.)

STEWED GREEN BURRITO

The bad news is that a burrito can potentially pack a day's worth of calories, saturated fats, and carbs all wrapped up in one. But the good news is that it absolutely doesn't have to. This vegetable lover's burrito is loaded with nutritiousness, deliciousness, and greenness, including green salsa, zucchini, lettuce, and herbs. In fact, it's so pleasingly stuffed that you shouldn't even try picking this one up. You'll save carb calories by not using an extra-large tortilla, too.

SERVES: 4 | SERVING SIZE: 1 burrito
PREP TIME: 20 minutes | COOK TIME: 24 minutes

- 1½ teaspoons avocado oil or peanut oil
- 2 medium zucchinis, unpeeled and finely chopped
- 1 small or ½ large yellow onion, finely chopped
- 2 large garlic cloves, minced
- ¾ cup medium tomatillo salsa (salsa verde)
- 1 (15-ounce) can no-salt-added pinto beans, drained (1½ cups)
- ⅛ teaspoon ground cumin, or to taste
- Pinch of sea salt (omit if you are following a sodium-modified eating plan)
- 1 teaspoon finely chopped fresh oregano leaves
- 3 tablespoons chopped fresh cilantro
- 4 (8-inch) whole-grain or grain-free tortillas of choice, warm
- ⅓ cup shredded plant-based Mexican- or Monterey Jack-style cheese*
- 2 cups packed shredded romaine lettuce (2 ounces)

**Note: Ideally, choose vegan cheese products based on tree nuts.*

DIRECTIONS

1. Heat the oil in a large stick-resistant skillet over medium-high heat. Add the zucchini and onion and sauté until the zucchini begins to caramelize and the onion is softened, about 5 minutes. Add the garlic and sauté until fragrant, about 1 minute. Add the salsa,

beans, cumin, and salt and stir for 1 minute to fully combine. Cover, reduce heat to low, and simmer until all the vegetables are fully softened, about 10 minutes.

2. Remove the lid, stir in the oregano, and continue to cook while stirring occasionally until no excess liquid remains, about 5 minutes. Stir in the cilantro. Adjust seasoning.
3. Onto each tortilla, sprinkle the cheese, bean mixture, and lettuce. Roll up tightly without folding in the ends. Secure closed with small bamboo picks, if desired. Enjoy with a fork and knife.

NUTRITION INFO

Choices/Exchanges: 2 starch, 2 vegetable, 1½ fat

Per Serving: 280 calories, 8 g total fat, 2 g saturated fat, 0 g trans fat, 0 mg cholesterol, 610 mg sodium, 781 mg potassium, 43 g total carbohydrate, 10 g dietary fiber, 7 g sugars, 0 g added sugars, 10 g protein, 139 mg phosphorus

How to Warm Tortillas

There are a few ways to warm your tortillas, which softens them up before use. Here are my two favorites. Heat a cast-iron skillet over medium-high and heat individual tortillas about 20 seconds per side. Or stack them up, fully wrap in unbleached parchment paper, and heat in the microwave for about 30 seconds. So easy.

NO-BRAINER BEAN BURRITO WRAP

If you like fast fixes for one, you're in luck. I intentionally crafted this Mexican-inspired wrap for use with convenient, yet nutrient-rich supermarket finds. When using convenience-style foods, keep it delicious and aim to keep all your picks free of artificial ingredients, added sugars, and excess sodium. I had all of that for this stuffed taco-style burrito recipe, which my friend Brian calls a burraco! It's also scrumptious when served as an overstuffed veggie burraco by adding leftover roasted or grilled veggies, like peppers or zucchini.

SERVES: 1 | SERVING SIZE: 1 wrap
PREP TIME: 5 minutes | COOK TIME: <1 minute

- 1 (8-inch) sprouted whole-grain or whole-wheat tortilla
- ¼ cup canned, lower-sodium, vegetarian refried beans
- ⅓ cup guacamole of choice (see recipes in this book)
- ½ cup packed, fresh, mixed salad greens
- ¼ cup deli-prepared pico de gallo or *Grape Tomato Pico de Gallo* (following recipe), drained of excess liquid
- Few drops hot sauce (optional)

DIRECTIONS

1. Place the tortilla on a microwave-safe plate. Using a spatula, spread the beans onto the tortilla, leaving about a 1-inch rim.
2. Heat in the microwave on high for 20 seconds or until warm.
3. While still warm, top with the guacamole, salad greens, and pico de gallo. Roll up or fold the tortilla over the fillings, add hot sauce if using, and serve.

NUTRITION INFO

Choices/Exchanges: 2½ starch, 1 vegetable, 1 lean protein, 2 fat

Per serving: 340 calories, 15 g total fat, 3.0 g saturated fat, 0 g trans fat, 0 mg cholesterol, 410 mg sodium, 1010 mg potassium, 45 g total carbohydrate, 12 g dietary fiber, 4 g sugars, 0 g added sugars, 11 g protein, 250 mg phosphorus

GRAPE TOMATO PICO DE GALLO

- 1 cup grape tomatoes, halved or quartered
- 1 scallion, green and white part, thinly sliced
- 1 tablespoon packed, small, fresh cilantro leaves
- 1 tablespoon lime juice
- ⅛ teaspoon sea salt

DIRECTIONS

In a medium bowl, stir together all ingredients. Serve, or store in a sealed jar or container in the refrigerator for up to 3 days. (Makes 4 servings, ¼ cup each.)

NUTRITION INFO

Choices/Exchanges = 0

Per serving: 10 calories, 0 g total fat, 0 g saturated fat, 0 g trans fat, 0 mg cholesterol, 70 mg sodium, 105 mg potassium, 2 g total carbohydrate, 1 g dietary fiber, 1 g sugars, 0 g added sugars, 0 g protein, 10 mg phosphorus

Almost Guacamole

Don't have guacamole on hand? Try my favorite version of "lazy" guacamole: Combine 1 diced Hass avocado, 3 tablespoons preservative-free salsa verde, and 2 tablespoons roughly chopped fresh cilantro leaves. That's it!

CHORIZO SEITAN AND VEGGIE TACOS

Chorizo is a well-seasoned pork sausage that you'll find in Mexican and Spanish cuisine. But there's definitely no pork here. Instead, you'll use chorizo-style seitan. Or, if you prefer, traditional seitan can be used—just sauté it in Step 2 along with a minced garlic clove, ½ teaspoon chili powder and/or cumin, and ½ teaspoon minced fresh oregano. Either way, seitan crumbles are sautéed along with cauliflower and kale to pump up the volume of this intriguing taco filling bursting with veggie goodness.

SERVES: 4 | SERVING SIZE: 2 tacos
PREP TIME: 12 minutes | COOK TIME: 12 minutes

- 1 tablespoon avocado oil or sunflower oil
- 3 cups small, bite-sized cauliflower florets (8 ounces)
- 8 ounces chorizo-style seitan, crumbled or finely chopped
- 2 scallions, thinly sliced, green and white parts separated
- 3 cups packed, chopped, fresh organic kale (2.5 ounces)
- Juice of 1 lime (2 tablespoons), divided
- ⅛ teaspoon sea salt, or to taste
- 8 small (5-inch) grain-free or whole-grain tortillas, gently warmed
- 3 tablespoons plant-based sour cream, or to taste

DIRECTIONS

1. In a large, deep, stick-resistant skillet or wok, heat the oil over medium-high heat. Add the cauliflower and sauté until it's lightly browned, about 3½ minutes.
2. Reduce heat to medium, add the seitan and white part of the scallions, and cook while stirring until the seitan is fully heated through, about 4 minutes. Add the kale, 1 tablespoon of the lime juice, and the salt, and cook while stirring until the kale is fully wilted, about 3 minutes. Stir in the remaining 1 tablespoon lime juice. Adjust seasoning.
3. Top tortillas with the seitan-veggie filling (⅓ rounded cup each), dollop with the plant-based sour cream, and sprinkle with the green part of the scallions. Fold and enjoy as tacos, with any additional desired toppings on the side.

NUTRITION INFO

Choices/Exchanges: 1½ starch, 1 vegetable, 2 very lean protein, 1 fat

Per serving: 270 calories, 8 g total fat, 1 g saturated fat, 0 g trans fat, 0 mg cholesterol, 560 mg sodium, 386 mg potassium, 30 g total carbohydrate, 5 g dietary fiber, 2 g sugars, 0 g added sugars, 21 g protein, 213 mg phosphorus

Plant-Based Taco Toppings

Keeping tacos simple can be scrumptious. But if you add toppings, they're definitely more fun. Plan to enjoy any of these toppings on these tacos and beyond for bonus fun: fresh avocado slices (my favorite!), guacamole or *Avocado Crema* (page 33), soft tree-nut cheese, small fresh cilantro sprigs, shredded purple cabbage or tricolor coleslaw mix, pepitas, pico de gallo, tomatillo or peach salsa, or lime zest.

Is Seitan a Soy Food?

Nope! Seitan is a wheat gluten food, not a soybean-based product. It has a meaty texture, which is why it works especially well as a stand-in for beef, chicken, or pork in stir-fried and sautéed dishes. In fact, its nickname is "wheat meat."

CHIMICHURRI HUMMUS AND CAULIFLOWER WRAP

Caramelized cauliflower is one of the key ingredients in this delightful entrée wrap. Don't worry, that doesn't mean it has caramel in it; "caramelized" is just a fancy-sounding culinary term that means browned. The other key is hummus, which goes beyond being a classic spread. It's transformed here into a full-flavored chimichurri-inspired hummus by way of parsley, oregano, garlic, vinegar, and hot pepper flakes. Paired with the veggies, it makes this a must-try wrap.

SERVES: 2 | SERVING SIZE: 1 wrap
PREP TIME: 18 minutes (not including hummus prep time) | COOK TIME: 8 minutes

- ½ cup hummus of choice (see recipes in this book)
- 2 tablespoons finely chopped fresh flat-leaf parsley
- 1 teaspoon finely chopped fresh oregano leaves
- 1 large garlic clove, minced
- 2 teaspoons extra-virgin olive oil, divided
- ½ teaspoon red wine vinegar
- ⅛ teaspoon freshly ground black pepper, or to taste
- ⅛ teaspoon dried hot pepper flakes, or to taste
- 2 cups small, bite-sized cauliflower florets
- ⅛ teaspoon sea salt, or to taste
- 2 (8-inch) whole-grain or flax tortillas or soft flatbreads of choice
- ¼ cup very thinly sliced red onion
- ⅔ cup cherry tomatoes, quartered

DIRECTIONS

1. Stir together the hummus, parsley, oregano, garlic, 1 teaspoon of the oil, the vinegar, black pepper, and hot pepper flakes until well-combined. Adjust seasoning. Set aside.
2. Heat the remaining 1 teaspoon oil in a large, stick-resistant skillet over medium-high heat. Add the cauliflower and salt, cover, and cook while shaking the pan or stirring occasionally until cooked through and well caramelized, about 7 minutes.
3. Spread the hummus over the entire surface of the tortillas. Sprinkle with the onion, cauliflower (preferably while warm), and tomatoes. Wrap and serve.

NUTRITION INFO

Choices/Exchanges: 2 starch, 1½ vegetable, 2 medium fat protein, 1½ fat

Per serving: 320 calories, 14 g total fat, 1.5 g saturated fat, 0 g trans fat, 0 mg cholesterol, 490 mg sodium, 520 mg potassium, 39 g total carbohydrate, 9 g dietary fiber, 5 g sugars, 0 g added sugars, 11 g protein, 250 mg phosphorus

Anytime Chimichurri Hummus

Beyond just slathering into this wrap, enjoy the chimichurri hummus whenever you're in the mood for a high-flavored dip or a twist on hummus. Just combine the first eight ingredients—hummus, parsley, oregano, garlic, olive oil, vinegar, black pepper, and hot pepper flakes. Go ahead and pick any hummus you like, even if you prefer a store-bought option.

HERB-ROASTED VEGETABLE WRAP

The rosemary-roasted mushrooms and bell peppers provide a sweet-savory pairing in this nourishing wrap that'll win over your appetite. The spread—which is a zingy mixture of hummus and balsamic vinegar—provides creaminess, tanginess, and full-bodied goodness. For easier eating after making the wraps, roll each up in unbleached parchment paper and peel down the paper as you bite into this bodacious delight. That's a wrap . . . a stuffed one!

SERVES: 2 | SERVING SIZE: 1 wrap
PREP TIME: 18 minutes (not including hummus prep time) | COOK TIME: 20 minutes

- 2 large portabella mushroom caps, sliced
- 2 medium bell peppers, preferably 1 red and 1 orange or yellow, sliced
- 2 large garlic cloves, minced
- 2 teaspoons avocado oil or extra-virgin olive oil
- ¾ teaspoon finely chopped fresh rosemary
- ¼ teaspoon freshly ground black pepper, or to taste
- ⅛ teaspoon sea salt, or to taste
- 3 tablespoons hummus of choice (see recipes in this book)
- 1 teaspoon aged balsamic vinegar
- 2 (8-inch) whole-wheat flour tortillas or grain-free tortillas
- 1 scallion, green and white parts, minced

DIRECTIONS

1. Preheat the oven to 450°F. In a large bowl, toss together the mushrooms, bell peppers, garlic, oil, rosemary, black pepper, and salt. Arrange in a single layer on a large silicone baking mat-lined baking sheet or unbleached parchment paper-lined baking sheet. Roast until the vegetables are fully cooked, about 20 minutes. (Note: Prepare in advance and chill, if desired.)
2. Mix together the hummus and balsamic vinegar in a small bowl until well-combined.
3. Spread the entire surface of each tortilla with the hummus mixture. Sprinkle each with the scallion and the roasted vegetables (warm or cool). Tightly roll up without tucking in sides.
4. Slice in half on the diagonal, and serve at room temperature.

NUTRITION INFO

Choices/Exchanges: 2 starch, 1 vegetable, 1 lean protein, 1 fat

Per serving: 260 calories, 10 g total fat, 2 g saturated fat, 0 g trans fat, 0 mg cholesterol, 570 mg sodium, 710 mg potassium, 36 g total carbohydrate, 8 g dietary fiber, 9 g sugars, 0 g added sugars, 9 g protein, 250 mg phosphorus

How to Buy and Store Portabella Mushrooms

Whether you're at a farmer's market or your local supermarket, choose portabella mushrooms that have a plump, smooth, and dry (but not overly dry) appearance. Simply put, they should look fresh. The rounded caps and the gills should seem firm, too.

If your mushrooms are packaged, store them the fridge in the original packaging. Otherwise, store them in a paper bag in the fridge. They'll ideally stay fresh in the refrigerator for up to a week.

If you don't need them within a week, prepare the portabellas and then you can freeze them for up to several weeks. Before prep, simply wipe them down with a slightly damp paper towel. And know that the full portabella is edible, including its gills and stem.

MAITAKE GYRO WITH MINTY TAHINI SAUCE

If the gyro used to be one of your go-to, late-night bites (it was for me in college!), you'll fully appreciate this diabetes-friendlier interpretation on it. I forgo the processed gyro meat in this 100-percent meat-free creation, and it has its own distinct and inviting taste. The sautéed maitake mushrooms are so savory and kind of meaty. The other unique addition is green tea, which makes the creamy tahini sauce saucy. Plus, when green tea is paired with starchy food, like pita bread, it may help prevent blood glucose spikes!

SERVES: 4 | SERVING SIZE: 1 gyro (½ stuffed pita pocket)
PREP TIME: 22 minutes | COOK TIME: 7 minutes

- ⅓ cup tahini
- ¼ cup unsweetened green or peppermint tea, chilled
- Juice of ½ small lemon (1 tablespoon), divided
- 1 small garlic clove, minced
- 1 teaspoon minced fresh mint
- ¼ teaspoon sea salt, divided
- 1 teaspoon extra-virgin olive oil
- 12 ounces fresh maitake mushrooms, separated, or sliced mushroom mixture
- 1 teaspoon finely chopped fresh oregano leaves
- 1 teaspoon freshly ground black pepper, or to taste
- 2 large whole-grain pitas, halved, warm
- 1 cup very thinly sliced, unpeeled, English cucumber
- 1 medium vine-ripened tomato, thinly sliced
- ⅓ cup extra-thinly sliced red onion

DIRECTIONS

1. With a fork, stir together the tahini, tea, ½ tablespoon of the lemon juice, the garlic, mint, and ⅛ teaspoon of the salt in a liquid measuring cup or small bowl until smooth. Adjust seasoning. Set aside.
2. Heat the oil in a large, stick-resistant skillet over medium-high heat. Add the mushrooms, oregano, pepper, and the remaining ⅛ teaspoon salt and sauté until the

mushrooms are fully softened and browned, about 6 minutes. Stir in the remaining ½ tablespoon lemon juice. Adjust seasoning.

3. Spoon half of the tahini sauce into the pita halves. Stuff with the cucumber, mushrooms, tomato, and onion. Serve with the remaining sauce on the side.

NUTRITION INFO

Choices/Exchanges: 1 starch, 1½ vegetable, 1 lean protein, 2 fat

Per serving: 260 calories, 13 g total fat, 2 g saturated fat, 0 g trans fat, 0 mg cholesterol, 310 mg sodium, 450 mg potassium, 32 g total carbohydrate, 7 g dietary fiber, 4 g sugars, 0 g added sugars, 9 g protein, 280 mg phosphorus

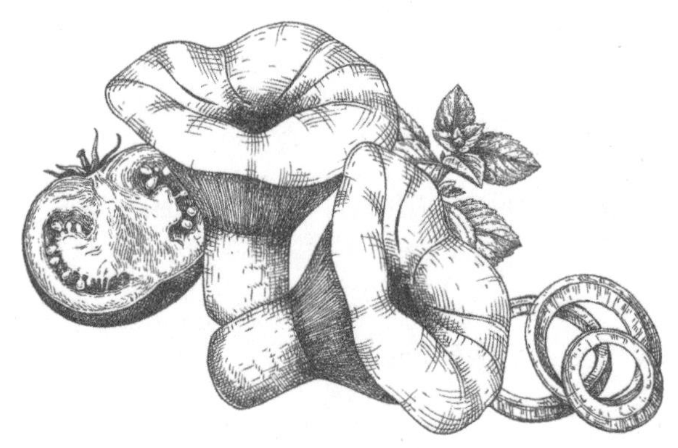

PORTABELLA BLT SANDWICH WITH HEIRLOOM TOMATOES

Have a hankering for a BLT sandwich? This plant-based version will satisfy your craving . . . and then some! The high-flavored, preservative-free *Smoky Portabella Bacon* is the perfect swap for the greasy, meaty strips. It has a bit of added sugar, but it comes naturally from diabetes-friendlier coconut sugar. And if you choose a tomato that's fully ripened and has never been refrigerated, you'll love sinking your teeth into the juicy, steak-like slices here. (Hint: This scrumptious sandwich is slightly high in sodium, so plan to keep sodium in check the rest of the day.)

SERVES: 4 | SERVING SIZE: 1 sandwich
PREP TIME: 7 minutes | COOK TIME: 5 minutes (when portabella bacon is prepared in advance)

- 8 slices whole-grain bread
- ¼ cup vegan mayo, aquafaba "mayo," or *Avocado Crema* (page 33)
- 1 recipe (48 strips) *Smoky Portabella Bacon* (page 79) or 4 servings vegan bacon of choice
- 2 cups packed (2 ounces) baby arugula or mixed baby salad greens
- 1 extra-large heirloom tomato, cut into 4 extra-thick slices

DIRECTIONS

1. Toast the bread.
2. Thinly spread the vegan mayo onto all of the toasts. Top four toasts with the portabella bacon, arugula, and tomatoes. Top with the remaining toasts, vegan mayo-side down.
3. Cut the sandwich in half using a bread knife. Enjoy!

NUTRITION INFO

Choices/Exchanges: 2 starch, 1 vegetable, 2 fat

Per serving: 280 calories, 12 g total fat, 2 g saturated fat, 0 g trans fat, 0 mg cholesterol, 740 mg sodium, 505 mg potassium, 34 g total carbohydrate, 2 g dietary fiber, 12 g sugars, 5 g added sugars, 9 g protein, 188 mg phosphorus

Vegan Bacon

Let's face it . . . processed meats, like bacon, are not health-conscious food picks for people with or at risk for diabetes. That's where vegan bacon comes in—whether homemade, like in this recipe, or store-bought. If you want to keep this sandwich as simple as possible, it's okay to buy ready-to-heat plant-based bacon. Most of the options available now are tastier and healthier than you might expect, though still processed. The best bets are generally tempeh or seitan bacon alternatives.

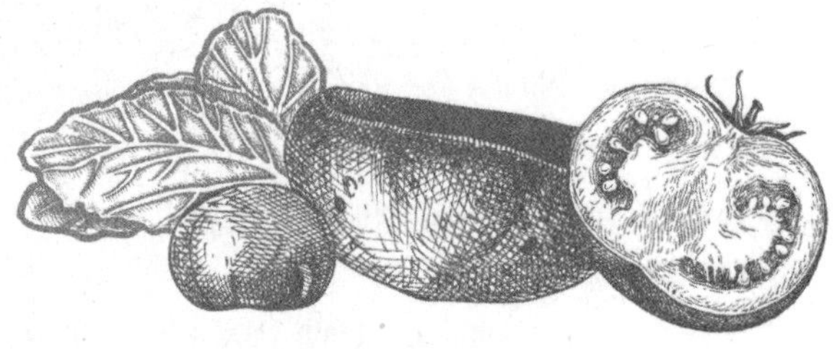

TAHINI CAESAR-STYLE SALAD WRAP WITH CRISPY CHICKPEAS

The refreshing Caesar-style salad that you'll make here tastes so much like the original version that's made with egg, Parmesan cheese, and anchovies, you'll surprise your taste buds—and everyone else's. But here, the dressing is based on tahini (sesame seed paste), lemon juice, lemon zest, green tea, olive oil and nutritional yeast flakes to create a memorably zingy taste. While you can stop there and munch on just the salad, you'll appreciate that it does double duty stuffed into tortillas and enjoyed by hand as a wrap. The roasted chickpeas (you can use the packaged variety) provide bonus crunch—no croutons required.

SERVES: 4 I SERVING SIZE: 1 wrap
PREP TIME: 22 minutes I COOK TIME: 0 minutes

- 1 recipe *Tahini Caesar-Style Dressing* (following recipe) or ½ cup bottled, plant-based Caesar dressing
- 8 ounces roughly chopped or torn romaine lettuce (about 1 head)
- 1½ tablespoons shelled hemp seeds or roasted sunflower seeds
- 4 (8-inch) whole-grain or grain-free tortillas or 4 *Fluffy Pulse-Based Flatbreads* (page 155)
- ½ cup crispy roasted chickpea or lentil snacks, such as *Wild Buffalo Chickpea Snackers* (page 55)
- ¼ teaspoon freshly ground black pepper (optional)

DIRECTIONS:

1. To a large mixing bowl, add the dressing and romaine lettuce and toss with tongs to combine. Sprinkle with the hemp seeds and toss to combine.
2. Top the tortillas with the salad, sprinkle with the chickpeas and, if using, the pepper.
3. Wrap each tortilla by folding up the bottom over the salad and folding in the sides, leaving the top open. Or enjoy open-face with a fork if using fluffy flatbread.

NUTRITION INFO

Choices/Exchanges: 2 starch, ½ high fat protein, 1½ fat

Per serving: 270 calories, 14 g total fat, 2.5 g saturated fat, 0 g trans fat, 0 mg cholesterol, 520 mg sodium, 457 mg potassium, 30 g total carbohydrate, 7 g dietary fiber, 3 g sugars, 0 g added sugars, 9 g protein, 138 mg phosphorus

Personalize It

Whether you enjoy this recipe as a wrap or you skip the tortilla and savor it as a salad, know that you can add your own twists to it. Want extra crunch? Sprinkle with toasted pine nuts or roasted pumpkin seeds. Want bonus zing? Stir drained capers, whole or chopped, into the dressing. Want to power-up the protein? Add just-baked, plant-based chicken tenders or nuggets.

TAHINI CAESAR-STYLE DRESSING

- 2 tablespoons tahini
- 1 teaspoon grated lemon zest
- Juice of ½ lemon (1½ tablespoons)
- 1½ tablespoons unsweetened jasmine green tea or other green tea, chilled
- 1 tablespoon extra-virgin olive oil
- 1 tablespoon nutritional yeast flakes
- 1 teaspoon Dijon mustard
- ½ teaspoon naturally brewed tamari or coconut aminos
- Few drops of vegan Worcestershire sauce
- 1 garlic clove, minced
- ¼ teaspoon sea salt, or to taste
- ¼ teaspoon coarsely ground black pepper, or to taste

In a mixing bowl, whisk together the tahini, lemon zest, lemon juice, tea, olive oil, nutritional yeast, mustard, tamari, Worcestershire sauce, garlic, salt, and pepper. (Makes about ½ cup dressing; 4 servings, 2 tablespoons each.)

NUTRITION INFO
Choices/Exchanges: 2 fat
Per serving: 90 calories, 8 g total fat, 1 g saturated fat, 0 g trans fat, 0 mg cholesterol, 210 mg sodium, 89 mg potassium, 3 g total carbohydrate, 1 g dietary fiber, 0 g sugars, 0 g added sugars, 3 g protein, 64 mg phosphorus

FLUFFY PULSE-BASED FLATBREAD

If you're looking for a homemade or grain-free flatbread, wrap, or tortilla, this easy recipe is my top pick. It's a simple stovetop twist on socca (farinata), which is a baked chickpea "pancake" from France. You can make it with endless delicious variations, too. Do use this chickpea flatbread throughout the recipes in this book—or with your other favorites—in place of tortillas, such as *Tahini Caesar-Style Salad Wrap with Crispy Chickpeas* (page 153). You can simply enjoy the flatbread as an anytime snack for just you, too. Multiply the recipe as you need.

SERVES: 1 | SERVING SIZE: 1 (7- to 8-inch) flatbread
PREP TIME: 8 minutes | COOK TIME: 4 minutes

- ¼ cup chickpea flour (30 grams)
- 3 tablespoons water
- ½ teaspoon extra-virgin olive oil
- ¼ teaspoon lemon juice
- ⅛ teaspoon baking soda or ¼ teaspoon ground chia seeds*
- Pinch of sea salt

DIRECTIONS:

1. In a small bowl or liquid measuring cup, whisk together all ingredients. (*For a fluffy flatbread, use baking soda; for a thinner tortilla/wrap, use ground chia seeds.) Let mixture stand for 5 minutes to allow ingredients to marry.
2. Meanwhile, preheat a medium cast-iron or other stick-resistant skillet over medium-high heat.
3. Pour and quickly spread the chickpea mixture into the skillet to form a 7- to 8-inch diameter round. Cook until golden brown on both sides and cooked through, about 1½ to 2 minutes per side. Serve.

NUTRITION INFO

Choices/Exchanges: 1 starch, ½ high fat protein

Per serving: 140 calories, 4.5 g total fat, 0.5 g saturated fat, 0 g trans fat, 0 mg cholesterol, 330 mg sodium, 256 mg potassium, 17 g total carbohydrate, 3 g dietary fiber, 3 g sugars, 0 g added sugars, 7 g protein, 96 mg phosphorus

Recipe Variations

Try this recipe with any mix-ins to the chickpea batter you like, ideally those that pair well with the toppings or fillings you plan to enjoy with this flatbread.

Herbal: Scallion + fresh rosemary + pinch of black pepper

Italian: Fresh basil leaves or basil pesto

Lebanese: Fresh mint leaves + pinch of garlic powder + pinch of cinnamon

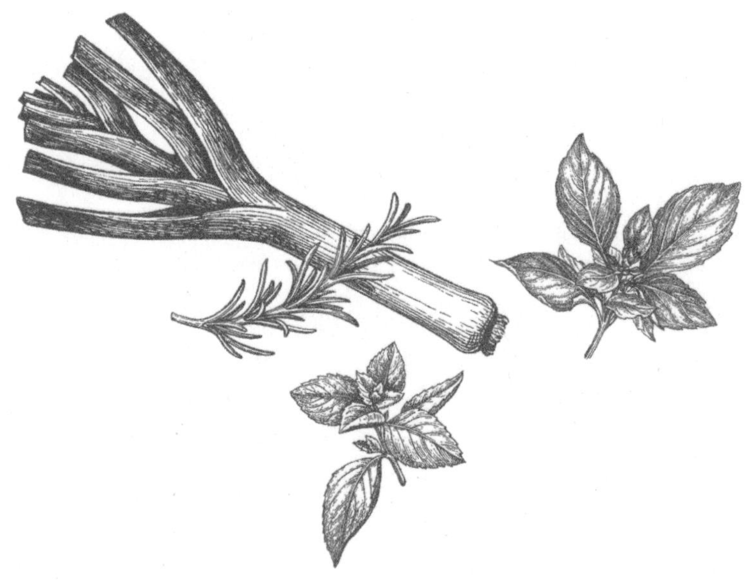

Bowls and Skillet Meals

SEASONAL VEGGIE POWER BOWL WITH THAI PEANUT DRESSING

With its plant protein and variety of nutrients, consider this a fresh, anytime entrée bowl, not a salad. Make it a colorful one by choosing eye-appealing veggies, like cucumber, carrot, and red bell pepper. Ideally pick what's available at a farmer's market to assure they're at their seasonal best. For a time-saver, both the dressing and edamame can be made in advance and chilled. For more nourishment, transform this into a power grain bowl by adding ½ cup of a chilled cooked grain, such as farro, bulgur, or brown rice, and serve with lime wedges on the side.

SERVES: 4 | SERVING SIZE: 2¾ cups
PREP TIME: 10 minutes (not including dressing prep) | COOK TIME: 8 minutes

- 1⅓ cups frozen, shelled, organic edamame
- ⅛ teaspoon sea salt
- 6 cups packed (6 ounces) mesclun or baby spring mix
- 3 cups thinly sliced or chopped seasonal veggies of choice or colorful bell peppers
- 4 servings (¾ cup) *Thai Peanut Dressing* (page 158)
- ¼ cup salted roasted peanuts
- ¼ cup packed fresh cilantro leaves or sliced Thai basil

DIRECTIONS

1. Prepare the edamame per package directions; drain, and sprinkle with the salt.
2. Arrange the mesclun, seasonal veggies, and prepared edamame into four bowls.
3. Drizzle the contents of each bowl with the *Thai Peanut Dressing;* sprinkle with the peanuts and cilantro, and serve.

NUTRITION INFO

Choices/Exchanges: 3 vegetable, 1 lean protein, 4 fat

Per serving: 310 calories, 21 g total fat, 3.5 g saturated fat, 0 g trans fat, 0 mg cholesterol, 450 mg sodium, 755 mg potassium, 16 g total carbohydrate, 7 g dietary fiber, 7 g sugars, 0 g added sugars, 15 g protein, 234 mg phosphorus

THAI PEANUT DRESSING

This dressing is so scrumptious, you'll want to enjoy it paired with lots of dishes. That's a good thing since this recipe makes 6 servings and you'll only need four servings of it for the *Seasonal Veggie Power Bowl with Thai Peanut Dressing*. With the rest, plan to enjoy this as a nutty dipping sauce for satay, basting sauce for grilled tofu, dressing for noodles, condiment for sandwiches, or drizzle sauce for roasted or grilled vegetables.

SERVES: 6 I SERVING SIZE: 3 tablespoons I PREP TIME: 10 minutes I COOK TIME: 0 minutes

- ½ cup creamy, natural, no-sugar-added peanut butter
- ⅓ cup plain, unsweetened coconut milk beverage (not canned coconut milk)
- 2 tablespoons unsweetened applesauce
- Juice of 1 lime (2 tablespoons)
- 1½ tablespoons naturally brewed soy sauce
- 1½ teaspoons freshly grated gingerroot
- 1 teaspoon toasted sesame oil
- ¼ teaspoon dried hot pepper flakes, or to taste

DIRECTIONS

Add the peanut butter, coconut milk beverage, applesauce, lime juice, soy sauce, ginger, sesame oil, and hot pepper flakes to a blender and purée. Store in a jar in the fridge for up to 1 week.

NUTRITION INFO

Choices/Exchanges: 1 high fat protein, 1 fat

Per serving: 150 calories, 13 g total fat, 2.5 g saturated fat, 0 g trans fat, 0 mg cholesterol, 290 mg sodium, 214 mg potassium, 4 g total carbohydrate, 2 g dietary fiber, 2 g sugars, 0 g added sugars, 6 g protein, 84 mg phosphorus

SCRAPPY BBQ BOWL

No, this entrée bowl isn't crappy. It's scrappy. And it'll make your taste buds 100-percent happy! In America, about 40 percent of our food is wasted. But it's absolutely possible to have great taste without waste. This bowl of yum offers a fantastic way to do that . . . by creatively using leftovers. Generally, the more mild-tasting the ingredients the better, so they'll work well together. Make this recipe with any food scraps you have on hand—or prepare it with super fresh ingredients when you don't have any ingredient odds and ends available. Either way, you'll finish the bowl in style with a tangy BBQ sauce, fresh cilantro, crunchy pepitas, and refreshing lime.

SERVES: 1 I SERVING SIZE: 1 bowl (about 3 cups)
PREP TIME: 10 minutes I COOK TIME: 1 minute, 15 seconds (if using precooked protein, veggies, and grains)

- 1½ cups packed fresh baby spinach
- 3 ounces large, bite-sized pieces of precooked, plant-based protein (such as baked organic tofu or plant-based "chicken"), chilled
- 1½ cups large, bite-sized pieces precooked, non-starchy veggies (such as grilled or roasted sweet bell peppers, broccoli, or zucchini), chilled
- ⅓ cup precooked quinoa or other whole-grains (such as farro or brown rice), chilled
- 2 tablespoons no-sugar-added barbecue sauce or *Fruit-Sweetened BBQ Sauce* (page 58)
- 2 tablespoons packed fresh cilantro leaves
- 2 tablespoons no-salt-added pepitas or sliced natural almonds
- 2 lime wedges

DIRECTIONS

1. Add the spinach to a microwave-safe bowl. Arrange the protein, veggies, and whole grains on top. Drizzle with the barbecue sauce.
2. Heat in the microwave on high for 1 minute, 15 seconds, or until hot. Adjust seasoning.
3. Sprinkle with the cilantro and pepitas. Serve with the lime wedges.

NUTRITION INFO
Choices/Exchanges: 1 starch, 4½ vegetable, 1½ very lean protein, 2 fat
Per serving: 340 calories, 13 g total fat, 2 g saturated fat, 0 g trans fat, 0 mg cholesterol, 430 mg sodium, 1197 mg potassium, 43 g total carbohydrate, 13 g dietary fiber, 5 g sugars, 0 g added sugars, 22 g protein, 448 mg phosphorus

On-the-Go Tip

For a take-to-work (or take-to-school) lunch, make your bowl and seal it tight at night. Grab and go in the morning and stash in the office fridge until ready for zapping in the microwave. Others will be envious!

Sauce Alternative

Give this bowl a worldly vibe. Instead of barbecue sauce, try salsa, *Thai Peanut Dressing,* (page 158) *Simple Lemony Tahini Sauce,* (page 104) or even a little bit of hot sauce. Switch up the citrus wedges as needed, such as using lemon wedges when using *Simple Lemony Tahini Sauce,* or even orange wedges when using *Thai Peanut Dressing.* There are endless possibilities!

PLANT-BASED BIBB AND BEAN BURRITO BOWL

If you've been thinking of beans as just a side dish, it's time to rethink. Eating beans every day may help people with type 2 diabetes better manage their blood glucose. So, consider regularly enjoying beans as the star of your entrée, like in this inviting meal-in-a-bowl that's full of health benefits. Enjoy all of this recipe's vivid colors, Mexican-inspired flavors, and lovely textures with a fork. The bowl itself is made from Bibb lettuce, so it's literally an edible bowl! But if you like, use the Bibb leaves to eat some of the bean mixture burrito style. Any way you choose to eat it, it's *muy delicioso.*

SERVES: 4 I SERVING SIZE: 1¾ cups
PREP TIME: 20 minutes I COOK TIME: 0 minutes

- 12 Bibb or Boston lettuce leaves
- 2½ cups cooked or drained canned beans, such as black, pinto, and/or kidney beans
- 2 cups grape tomatoes, quartered lengthwise
- 1¼ cups frozen corn, thawed
- 3 scallions, green and white parts, very thinly sliced on diagonal
- ⅓ cup finely diced, plant-based, Monterey Jack-style cheese or crumbled, plant-based, feta-style cheese* (1½ ounces)
- ¼ cup chopped fresh cilantro
- ¼ teaspoon ground cumin, or to taste
- ¼ teaspoon chili powder, or to taste
- ¼ teaspoon sea salt, or to taste
- 1 Hass avocado, peeled, pitted, and diced
- ⅔ cup medium or "hot" tomatillo salsa (salsa verde)
- 4 lime wedges

**Note: Ideally, choose vegan cheese products based on tree nuts.*

DIRECTIONS

1. Divide the lettuce leaves among 4 dinner plates or pasta bowls, loosely forming a "bowl" with the leaves.

2. Stir together the beans, tomatoes, corn, scallions, plant-based cheese, cilantro, cumin, chili powder, and salt in a medium bowl. Add the avocado and salsa and gently stir just to combine. Adjust seasoning.
3. Evenly divide the bean mixture among the 4 lettuce "bowls," and serve with the lime wedges on the side.

NUTRITION INFO

Choices/Exchanges: 2 starch, 2 vegetable, 1½ fat

Per serving: 300 calories, 9 g total fat, 1 g saturated fat, 0 g trans fat, 0 mg cholesterol, 480 mg sodium, 1137 mg potassium, 48 g total carbohydrate, 14 g dietary fiber, 6 g sugars, 0 g added sugars, 12 g protein, 242 mg phosphorus

How to Prepare Dry Beans

Canned beans are super convenient. When using them, I suggest selecting an organic variety so all that's in the can are the nourishing beans, water, and sometimes salt or sea salt. However, if you prefer to use dried beans, here's how to prepare them:

Rinse 1 pound beans well and discard any stones. Add the beans and 10 to 12 cups water to a large pot or bowl. Refrigerate overnight or about 8 hours. Drain, rinse the beans, and return the beans to the large pot. Cover the beans with about 3 inches of water (add more water during cooking, if necessary). Bring to a boil. Then, reduce the heat to low and simmer uncovered, stirring occasionally, until tender, about 1 hour and 15 minutes (cooking time may vary). Drain beans and use in recipes or add the beans to ice cold water until just cool, drain well, and freeze in 1- or 1½-cup packages. Makes about 5 cups cooked beans.

CARIBBEAN BLACK BEAN BOWL

If you appreciate exploring global cuisine, you'll adore the worldly flavor appeal of this bowl recipe. You'll prepare it like a stir-fry, but it has nothing to do with Chinese takeout! All of the tastes and textures of this vivid recipe work so well together. The coconut milk creates richness and a distinct Caribbean accent. Once you prep the ingredients, this "stir-fry" is so quick to fix. Serve as is or try over steamed brown jasmine rice for a complete meal in a bowl that tastes rather tropical.

SERVES: 4 | SERVING SIZE: 1⅓ cups
PREP TIME: 20 minutes | COOK TIME: about 12 minutes

- 1 tablespoon avocado oil or peanut oil
- 1 large sweet potato, scrubbed, unpeeled, finely diced
- 2 large green bell peppers, diced
- 2 teaspoons freshly grated gingerroot
- 2 large garlic cloves, very thinly sliced
- 3 scallions, thinly sliced, green and white parts separated
- 1 (15-ounce) can black beans, gently rinsed and drained (1½ cups)
- 1 cup small grape tomatoes
- ½ cup low-sodium vegetable broth
- ½ cup light organic (canned) coconut milk
- ½ teaspoon sea salt, or to taste
- ⅛ teaspoon ground cayenne or black pepper, or to taste
- Pinch of ground cinnamon or allspice, or to taste
- 2 tablespoons coarsely chopped, roasted, unsalted peanuts

DIRECTIONS

1. Heat the oil in a wok or large skillet over high heat. Add the sweet potato and stir-fry for 2 minutes. Add the bell peppers and stir-fry until the sweet potato and bell peppers are caramelized, about 5 minutes. Add the ginger, garlic, and white part of the scallions and stir-fry for 30 seconds. Add the beans, tomatoes, broth, coconut milk, salt, cayenne, and cinnamon and stir-fry until the excess liquid has evaporated yet mixture is still very

moist, about 2½ to 3 minutes. Stir in the green part of the scallions. Remove from heat. Adjust seasoning.

2. Transfer to a large serving bowl or individual bowls, sprinkle with the peanuts, and serve.

NUTRITION INFO

Choices/Exchanges: 2 starch, 1 vegetable, 1 fat

Per serving: 230 calories, 8 g total fat, 2 g saturated fat, 0 g trans fat, 0 mg cholesterol, 460 mg sodium, 850 mg potassium, 34 g total carbohydrate, 9 g dietary fiber, 11 g sugars, 0 g added sugars, 8 g protein, 190 mg phosphorus

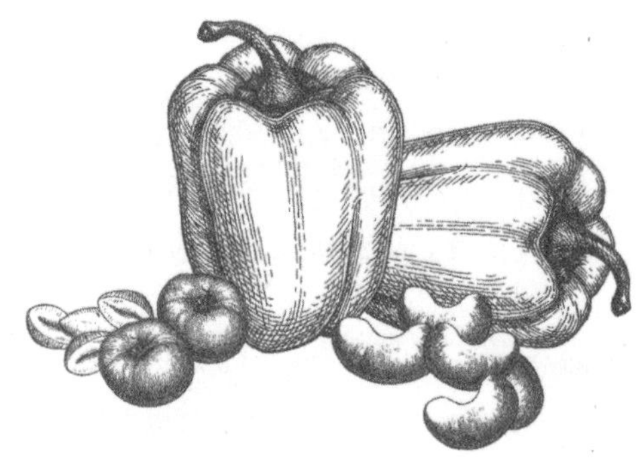

CAJUN GRAIN MINI-BOWL

Served as a right-sized entrée or generous side, this scrumptious whole-grain dish is inspired by classic "dirty" rice. You can also consider it a twist on red beans and rice. Thank you, Louisiana! Here, the stars are red beans and farro. The soluble fiber-filled kidney beans may help manage blood glucose levels. And it tastes like the beans have been simmered for hours. The plant-based "meat" or seitan provides meatiness without meat. And if you're not a plant-based "meat" or seitan aficionado, swap chopped baby bellas (crimini mushrooms) in its place in Step 2. Either way, this full-flavored Cajun dish is a bowl of delish.

SERVES: 6 | SERVING SIZE: about 1 cup
PREP TIME: 16 minutes | COOK TIME: 40 to 45 minutes

- 1 cup uncooked whole (regular) farro, rinsed and drained
- 1¾ cups low-sodium vegetable broth
- 1 (14.5-ounce) can roasted, diced tomatoes with green chilies (do not drain)
- 1 teaspoon sea salt, or to taste
- ½ teaspoon freshly ground black pepper, or to taste
- 1 tablespoon extra-virgin olive oil
- 5 ounces uncooked, non-GMO, plant-based ground "meat" or finely chopped seitan
- 1 large green bell pepper, finely diced
- 1 small white onion, finely diced
- 1 tablespoon salt-free Cajun seasoning, or to taste (see *Cajun Changin'* on the following page)
- 1 (15-ounce) can no-salt-added red kidney beans, drained

DIRECTIONS

1. Add the farro, broth, diced tomatoes with liquid, salt, and pepper to a large saucepan. Bring to a boil over high heat. Reduce the heat to medium low, cover, and simmer for 20 minutes. (The farro will be about halfway cooked.)

2. Meanwhile, heat the oil in a large stick-resistant skillet over medium-high heat. Add the "meat," bell pepper, onion, and Cajun seasoning and sauté until mixture is lightly browned, about 7 minutes.
3. Stir the "meat" mixture and beans into the farro mixture, cover, and simmer over low until the farro is tender, about 15 to 20 minutes.
4. Remove from heat and let stand, covered, for 5 minutes to complete the cooking process. Adjust seasoning. Then serve in bowls.

NUTRITION INFO

Choices/Exchanges: 3 starch, 1 lean protein

Per serving: 300 calories, 7 g total fat, 1.5 g saturated fat, 0 g trans fat, 0 mg cholesterol, 695 mg sodium, 676 mg potassium, 44 g total carbohydrate, 9 g dietary fiber, 4 g sugars, 0 g added sugars, 15 g protein, 107 mg phosphorus

Cajun Changin'

If your palate enjoys mild instead of more wild flavors, simply use a little less Cajun seasoning. You can always add more seasoning at the end of cooking if you want more kick. But if you're not able to find salt-free Cajun seasoning, you can make your own. Mix together ½ teaspoon each of sweet paprika, garlic powder, onion powder, cayenne pepper, dried thyme or oregano, and freshly ground black pepper. (Makes 1 tablespoon seasoning.)

SAUCY PEANUT SOBA NOODLES WITH SLAW

If you need a new go-to recipe for a quick lunch, try this. It's one of my regulars. The recipe is based on 100 percent buckwheat soba noodles, which only take about 8 minutes (or less!) to cook. By the way, buckwheat isn't related to wheat; it's a seed of a flowering plant that's a good source of protein and contains the antioxidants rutin and quercetin. And that's good news for your health. As for the taste of the finished noodle dish . . . it's really saucy and downright craveable! You'll love that you can just toss in premade coleslaw mix to further punch up the nutrition and crunch of this pan-Asian-inspired cool fix.

SERVES: 4 | SERVING SIZE: 1½ cups
PREP TIME: 8 minutes | COOK TIME: 10 minutes

- 8 cups cold water
- ¼ cup creamy, natural, no-sugar-added peanut butter
- ¼ cup unsweetened applesauce
- ¼ cup rice or brown rice vinegar
- 2 tablespoons reduced-sodium tamari (soy sauce)
- 6 ounces dry 100% buckwheat soba noodles or dry whole-wheat spaghetti
- 4 cups fresh coleslaw mix (about 10 ounces)
- ¼ cup packed fresh cilantro leaves
- 4 lime wedges (optional)

DIRECTIONS

1. Add water to a large saucepan and bring to a boil over high heat.
2. While the water is coming to a boil, whisk together the peanut butter, applesauce, vinegar, and soy sauce until smooth in a large mixing bowl. Set aside.
3. Using tongs, stir the noodles into the boiling water and cook according to package directions, about 8 minutes. Drain the noodles using a strainer. Rinse noodles with cold water (or toss with ice cubes) to cool; drain again.
4. Transfer the noodles to the large bowl with the peanut butter sauce. Toss with tongs to combine. Add the coleslaw mix and cilantro, and toss with tongs to combine. If desired, garnish with a little additional cilantro and squeeze a lime wedge over top. Serve.

NUTRITION INFO

Choices/Exchanges: 2½ starch, 1 vegetable, 1½ fat

Per serving: 290 calories, 10 g total fat, 1.4 g saturated fat, 0 g trans fat, 0 mg cholesterol, 270 mg sodium, 480 mg potassium, 44 g total carbohydrate, 6 g dietary fiber, 5 g sugars, 0 g added sugars, 9 g protein, 245 mg phosphorus

Go Confetti Style

Instead of slaw mix based on green cabbage, choose a tricolor blend. Or go DIY by tossing together 2 cups of shredded green cabbage, 1½ cups of shredded purple cabbage, and ½ cup of shredded carrot. If you're a broccoli lover, try this with broccoli slaw instead. For an herbal twist, occasionally finish with mint or basil leaves rather than cilantro. And to transform into a protein-packed pick, toss in roasted peanuts or baked tofu cubes—or both!

SKILLET BEANS AND GREENS WITH COCONUTTY RICED CAULIFLOWER

This recipe proves that easy and tasty can absolutely go together. You'll wonder what took you so long to discover this palate-pleasing, plant-based dinner for two. The double whammy of fiber and protein makes it quite satisfying. And the mixture of spices in the skillet-cooked beans and greens, along with coconut milk-spiked riced cauliflower, takes it over the top flavor-wise. Now that you've discovered the recipe, go stock up on garbanzo beans—and all of the other pantry staples in the ingredient list.

SERVES: 2 | SERVING SIZE: 2½ cups
PREP TIME: 12 minutes | COOK TIME: 6 minutes (does not include precooking time for *Caramelized Riced Cauliflower)*

- 1 recipe cooked *Caramelized Riced Cauliflower* (page 215) or 2 cups cooked riced vegetable of choice, chilled
- 3 tablespoons light organic (canned) coconut milk
- 1 tablespoon extra-virgin olive oil
- 1 (15-ounce) can no-salt-added chickpeas (garbanzo beans), drained (do not rinse)
- 1 teaspoon curry powder
- ½ teaspoon ground ginger
- ¼ teaspoon freshly ground black pepper
- 1 (5-ounce) package fresh baby spinach
- ¼ teaspoon sea salt
- 3 tablespoons fresh cilantro leaves

DIRECTIONS

1. In a medium saucepan, add the chilled riced cauliflower and coconut milk. Cook while stirring over medium-high heat until steamy, about 3 minutes. Then reduce heat to low, cover, and keep warm.
2. Meanwhile, in a large skillet, heat the olive oil over medium heat. Add the garbanzo beans, curry powder, ginger, and pepper, and stir to coat. Add the spinach and salt, and cook while gently stirring until the beans are heated through and the spinach is just wilted, about 2½ minutes.

3. In individual bowls, top the riced cauliflower with the beans and greens, sprinkle with the cilantro leaves, and serve.

NUTRITION INFO
Choices/Exchanges: 2½ starch, 1 vegetable, 1½ fat
Per serving: 340 calories, 15 g total fat, 2.5 g saturated fat, 0 g trans fat, 0 mg cholesterol, 530 mg sodium, 1044 mg potassium, 41 g total carbohydrate, 15 g dietary fiber, 6 g sugars, 0 g added sugars, 14 g protein, 246 mg phosphorus

A Spice with Benefits

Curcumin is a natural compound in turmeric. And turmeric is a spice found in curry powder. The compound provides a distinctive golden-yellow color and has shown potential for lowering blood glucose levels. So keep curry powder or turmeric near your salt and pepper shakers to remember to sprinkle it onto dishes more regularly.

SZECHWAN TEMPEH GREENMARKET SKILLET

Ready to go to the farmer's market? If so, peruse the ingredients list and pick up all of the produce for this skillet recipe, even if you make a few personalized veggie changes. The recipe easily lends itself to seasonal swaps. Once home, celebrate your farmer's market haul by fixing this. Unlike if you order takeout, here you'll know exactly what you're getting. Stir-frying offers a simple, quick, and tasty way to get plenty of vegetables into your meal, too. I suggest cooking the rice or other whole grain in advance. Then you can just focus on making the stir-fry at mealtime.

SERVES: 4 I SERVING SIZE: 2 cups
PREP TIME: 15 minutes I COOK TIME: 10 minutes (plus rice cooking time)

- ¾ cup low-sodium vegetable broth
- ¼ cup fruit-sweetened or no-sugar-added ketchup
- 2 tablespoons naturally brewed soy sauce, or to taste
- 1½ tablespoons Asian garlic-chili sauce
- 1½ teaspoons grated fresh gingerroot
- 1 tablespoon toasted sesame oil
- 8 ounces organic tempeh, cut into 24 pieces
- ½ large Vidalia or other sweet onion, sliced
- 3 cups bite-sized broccoli florets (8 ounces)
- 2 large red bell peppers, sliced, or 3 cups bite-sized cauliflower florets
- 2 cups steamed brown basmati rice or cooked whole-grain of choice, warm*
- ¼ cup pine nuts, pan-toasted, or chopped unsalted, roasted peanuts
- 1 scallion, green part only, thinly sliced

***Tip:** *Make the rice in advance and, if needed, reheat.*

DIRECTIONS

1. In a small saucepan over medium-high heat, add the broth, ketchup, soy sauce, chili sauce, and ginger. Cook for 5 minutes, stirring occasionally.

2. Meanwhile, heat the oil in an extra-large cast-iron or other stick-resistant skillet over medium-high heat. (Reduce the heat if the oil begins to smoke.) Stir-fry the tempeh and onion until the tempeh is lightly browned, about 5 minutes. Add the broccoli and bell peppers and stir-fry for 2 minutes.
3. Add the broth mixture and continue to stir-fry until vegetables are tender-crisp, about 1 minute.
4. Push the stir-fry to one half of the skillet and add the prepared rice to the other half. Sprinkle everything with the pine nuts and scallion and serve from the skillet. If desired, serve with additional soy sauce on the side.

NUTRITION INFO

Choices/Exchanges: 2 starch, 2 vegetable, 1 very lean protein, 3 fat

Per serving: 390 calories, 17 g total fat, 2.5 g saturated fat, 0 g trans fat, 0 mg cholesterol, 670 mg sodium, 826 mg potassium, 45 g total carbohydrate, 5 g dietary fiber, 9 g sugars, 0 g added sugars, 19 g protein, 388 mg phosphorus

What Is Tempeh?

Tempeh is a fermented soybean cake. It looks a little like a weird, crispy-rice cereal treat. But it's the type of cake that's savory, not sweet. With its dense, chewy texture, it works well in place of meat in this stir-fry. And with its chameleon-like ability to take on taste, the Asian flavors will shine through. Look for it in the refrigerated section of the grocery store.

CHICK'N AND ZUCCHINI PARMESAN IN A PAN

Looking for a special occasion dish? Here you go! This indulgent "chicken" parm is based on breaded vegan "chicken" patties and embraces plant-based cheese. And it's simple to fix. Look for cashew or other tree nut-based, plant-based cheese for the most nourishing choice. You'll love this over the ribbons of zucchini—or, if you prefer, call them zoodles. Altogether, this skillet main dish is absolutely scrumptious. *Mangia, mangia!*

SERVES: 4 | SERVING SIZE: ¼ of skillet with 1 "chicken" patty
PREP TIME: 15 minutes | COOK TIME: 19 to 20 minutes

- 4 (2.5-ounce) frozen, breaded, plant-based "chicken" patties
- ½ teaspoon dry no-salt-added Italian seasoning
- 2 tablespoons extra-virgin olive oil
- 2 medium (8- to 9-ounce) zucchini, shredded into long fettuccine-like strands with a vegetable peeler, or 16 ounces fresh spiralized zucchini
- Pinch of sea salt
- ¾ cup no-sugar-added marinara or arrabbiata sauce of choice
- 2 tablespoons grated vegan Parmesan-style cheese*
- 4 ounces plant-based fresh Italian-style mozzarella cheese, thinly sliced*
- ¼ cup packed fresh basil leaves, torn

**Note: Ideally, choose vegan cheese products based on tree nuts.*

DIRECTIONS

1. Prepare the plant-based "chicken" patties per package directions. Sprinkle with the Italian seasoning and set aside.
2. Heat the olive oil in a large (12-inch) cast-iron or other stick-resistant skillet over medium heat. Add the zucchini and salt and cook while tossing occasionally with tongs until the zucchini is slightly softened, about 3 minutes.
3. Nestle the prepared plant-based patties onto the zucchini. On top of the patties, evenly spoon the marinara sauce, sprinkle with vegan parmesan, and top with the plant-based

mozzarella. Note: If you're on a sodium-modified eating plan, use a low-sodium marinara sauce.

4. Cover and cook until the cheese is melted and zucchini is golden brown on the bottom, about 4 to 5 minutes. Sprinkle with the basil and serve from the skillet.

NUTRITION INFO

Choices/Exchanges: 1 starch, 2 vegetable, 1 medium fat protein, 3 fat

Per serving: 330 calories, 21 g total fat, 7 g saturated fat, 0 g trans fat, 0 mg cholesterol, 750 mg sodium, 467 mg potassium, 25 g total carbohydrate, 2 g dietary fiber, 6 g sugars, 0 g added sugars, 14 g protein, 160 mg phosphorus

Cooking for One or Two?

You're in luck if you prefer to make this Italian-inspired dish when dining solo or as a couple. It'll work equally well for you and is easily adjustable. First, divide ingredient amounts by four (for one person) or by two (for two people). Then, ideally use a smaller skillet: 8-inch pan (for one person) or 10-inch pan (for two people).

Salads: Bean, Grain, and Leafy Greens

BLACK BEAN AND AVOCADO COBB SALAD WITH CARROT VINAIGRETTE

It's been around since 1937, but the Cobb salad is still a delight today. And it's especially delightful in this loosely-inspired, contemporary makeover of the classic version. As you dig your fork into this salad bowl, you'll experience the culinary excitement of an array of veggie textures, colors, and tastes arranged atop a bed of mesclun. Avocado is included for lusciousness. Beans make it hearty and punch up its protein. And to top that off, the tarragon-laced carrot vinaigrette is uniquely delicious and makes this Cobb-style salad no run-of-the-mill recipe.

SERVES: 4 | SERVING SIZE: about 2½ cups
PREP TIME: 18 minutes | COOK TIME: 0 minutes

- 5 cups packed mesclun or baby spring mix (5 ounces)
- 1 cup grape tomatoes, halved lengthwise
- ½ cup finely diced red onion
- ¼ cup sun-dried tomato bits, not oil-packed (rehydrated, if necessary)

- 1 (15-ounce) can black or kidney beans, gently rinsed and drained (1½ cups)
- 1 Hass avocado, peeled, pitted, diced
- 1 ounce white button mushrooms, fresh or grilled, thinly sliced
- 1 recipe (about ½ cup) *Carrot Vinaigrette* (see the following)
- ¼ teaspoon sea salt, or to taste
- ½ teaspoon freshly ground black pepper, or to taste
- 1 lime, cut into wedges

DIRECTIONS

1. Arrange the mesclun on four plates. Top with the grape tomatoes, onion, sun-dried tomato bits, black beans, avocado, and mushrooms.
2. Drizzle the *Carrot Vinaigrette* over the salad, sprinkle with the salt and pepper, and serve with the lime wedges.

NUTRITION INFO

Choices/Exchanges: 1 starch, 1½ vegetable, 2 fat

Per serving: 210 calories, 9 g total fat, 1.5 g saturated fat, 0 g trans fat, 0 mg cholesterol, 370 mg sodium, 820 mg potassium, 27 g total carbohydrate, 9 g dietary fiber, 7 g sugars, 0 g added sugars, 8 g protein, 170 mg phosphorus

CARROT VINAIGRETTE

- ¼ cup pure-pressed carrot juice
- Juice of 1 lime (2 tablespoons)
- 1 tablespoon extra-virgin olive oil
- 1 tablespoon finely chopped fresh tarragon or cilantro
- ⅛ teaspoon sea salt

DIRECTIONS

Whisk together all ingredients in a liquid measuring cup or small bowl. (Makes about ½ cup; 4 servings, about 2 tablespoons each.)

NUTRITION INFO

Choices/Exchanges: 1 fat

Per serving: 40 calories, 3.5 g total fat, 0 g saturated fat, 0 g trans fat, 0 mg cholesterol, 85 mg sodium, 59 mg potassium, 2 g total carbohydrate, 0 g dietary fiber, 1 g sugars, 0 g added sugars, 0 g protein, 8 mg phosphorus

TARRAGON WHITE BEAN SALAD

I often get asked about simple ways to get enough protein on a plant-based diet. And one of my many responses is to plan more beans into meals. Since canned cannellini beans are a key pantry staple, you're just seven minutes away from more protein if you plan this recipe into your repertoire. Plus, beans' duo of protein and fiber make them especially satiating. The addition of fresh tarragon makes this simply prepared recipe special.

SERVES: 3 I SERVING SIZE: ½ cup
PREP TIME: 7 minutes I COOK TIME: 0 minutes

- 1½ tablespoons white balsamic or white wine vinegar
- 1½ tablespoons extra-virgin olive oil
- 1 teaspoon Dijon mustard
- 1 teaspoon finely chopped fresh tarragon
- ⅛ teaspoon freshly ground black pepper, or to taste
- 1 (15-ounce) can cannellini or other white beans, gently rinsed and drained (1½ cups)
- 1 small shallot, minced
- 3 tablespoons finely diced celery or fennel (optional)

DIRECTIONS

1. Whisk together the vinegar, oil, mustard, tarragon, and pepper in a medium bowl. Add the beans, shallot and, if using, celery and toss to combine.
2. Serve in individual bowls. Garnish, if desired, with additional fresh tarragon leaves.

NUTRITION INFO

Choices/Exchanges: 1½ starch, 1 lean protein

Per serving: 190 calories, 7 g total fat, 1 g saturated fat, 0 g trans fat, 0 mg cholesterol, 400 mg sodium, 500 mg potassium, 24 g total carbohydrate, 7 g dietary fiber, 4 g sugars, 0 g added sugars, 9 g protein, 100 mg phosphorus

CANNELLINI BEAN VERSATILITY

Cannellini beans are quite versatile in cuisine. They can be blended into recipes to provide creaminess without cream, like in an Italian vodka sauce or *Roasted Orange Bell Pepper Soup.* (page 247) Of course, they can be sensational in a starring role, like in this bean salad, *Tuscan Vegetable Stew,* (page 255) *California Cannellini Chili,* (page 259) and *Lemony White Bean and Rosemary Crostini.* (page 51).

Also consider using cannellini beans as a simple swap for other varieties to bring new culinary interest to a recipe. For instance, whirl up a hummus with white beans instead of chickpeas; make a chili with them in place of red kidney beans; or create refried cannellini beans instead of using traditional pinto or black beans.

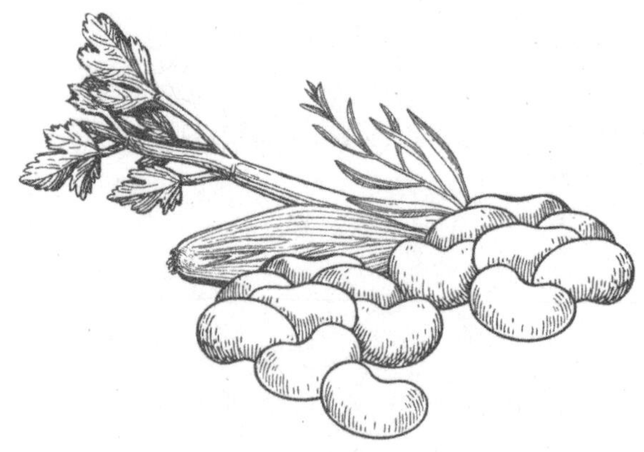

FRENCH LENTIL SALAD

Chickpeas (garbanzo beans) seem to be getting a majority of the pulse family love these days. But lentils deserve the spotlight, too. So show them off! Make this lemony dressed lentil salad when you need a satisfying side. It's got such appealing texture. The duo of carrots and dill is a highlight, and the combination of 8 grams of plant protein and 8 grams of dietary fiber is so satisfying. Since this is no wimpy salad, it keeps well in the fridge for several days. Plan it into a couple meals—or even enjoy as a stand-alone snack!

SERVES: 6 | SERVING SIZE: ⅔ cup salad
PREP TIME: 8 minutes | COOK TIME: 30 minutes (plus cooling time)

- 1 cup dry French green lentils, rinsed and drained
- 1 (32-fluid-ounce) carton low-sodium vegetable broth
- Juice of 1 lemon (3 tablespoons)
- 1 tablespoon extra-virgin olive oil
- ½ teaspoon sea salt
- 1 cup shredded carrots
- ¼ cup packed fresh dill fronds (feathery leaves)

DIRECTIONS

1. In a large saucepan, add the lentils and broth. Bring to a boil over high heat. Reduce heat to medium low and simmer, partially covered, until the lentils are tender, about 25 minutes. Drain any excess broth.
2. In a large bowl, whisk together the lemon juice, oil, and salt. Add the hot lentils (do not rinse) and the carrots and stir to combine. Set aside to cool for about 30 minutes. Stir, then chill in the refrigerator until ready to serve.
3. Stir the dill into the lentil salad just before serving.

NUTRITION INFO
Choices/Exchanges: 1 starch, 1 vegetable, 1 lean protein
Per serving: 140 calories, 2.5 g total fat, 0.4 g saturated fat, 0 g trans fat, 0 mg cholesterol, 270 mg sodium, 440 mg potassium, 21 g total carbohydrate, 8 g dietary fiber, 4 g sugars, 0 g added sugars, 8 g protein, 195 mg phosphorus

GOT EXTRA BROTH?

In this recipe, you'll drain any excess broth used for lentil preparation. When you have extra broth, make a plan for it. Perhaps drizzle it over other meal components for extra scrumptiousness. Otherwise, cool it, then freeze it in ice cube trays. Once frozen, store the broth cubes in a freezer container for later use, such as plopping into the cooking liquid for whole grains.

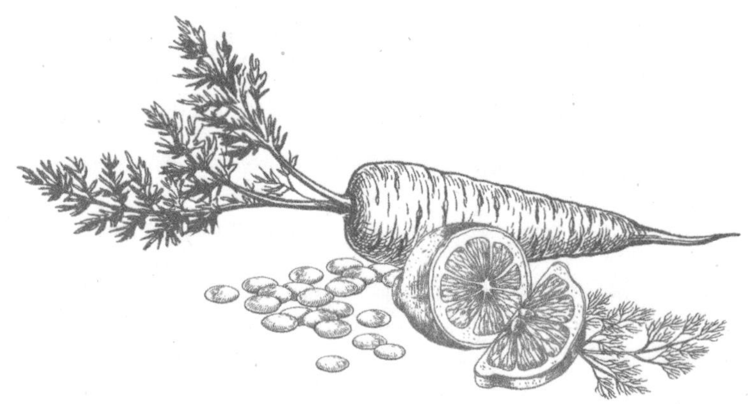

GRILLED ASPARAGUS SPEARS SALAD

What's your favorite vegetable? Frankly, I don't know if I have just one, but asparagus is up there. I'm completely enamored by grilled asparagus. I indulge on spears like French fries . . . no ketchup, of course! Here they transform a simple salad into one that's wow-worthy. The lemony vinaigrette brings it all together in perfect culinary harmony. If you pick up the asparagus spears from this salad with your fingers, I promise I won't tell anyone! Using a fork and a knife is more polite, of course.

SERVES: 4 | SERVING SIZE: 1½ cups salad with 6 asparagus spears
PREP TIME: 10 minutes | COOK TIME: 8 to 10 minutes

- 24 asparagus spears, ends trimmed
- 1½ tablespoon extra-virgin olive oil, divided
- ⅛ teaspoon sea salt, or to taste
- Juice of 1 small lemon (2 tablespoons)
- 6 cups packed mesclun or baby spring mix (6 ounces)
- 2 tablespoons thinly sliced fresh basil
- ⅓ cup finely diced red onion, divided
- ¼ teaspoon freshly ground black pepper, or to taste

DIRECTIONS

1. Prepare an outdoor or indoor grill. Place the asparagus into a 9- by 13-inch or similar-sized dish, sprinkle with ½ tablespoon of the oil and the salt and toss to coat.
2. Grill the asparagus (in batches, if necessary) until lightly charred and just tender over medium-high heat, turning only as needed, about 8 to 10 minutes.
3. Meanwhile, whisk together the lemon juice with the remaining 1 tablespoon oil in a large bowl. Add the mesclun, basil, and half of the onion and toss to coat. If desired, add a pinch of salt, to taste. Arrange the mesclun salad on individual plates.
4. Top each salad with 6 of the grilled asparagus spears. Sprinkle with the remaining onion and the pepper and serve.

NUTRITION INFO
Choices/Exchanges: 2 vegetable, 1 fat
Per serving: 80 calories, 5 g total fat, 1 g saturated fat, 0 g trans fat, 0 mg cholesterol, 90 mg sodium, 340 mg potassium, 7 g total carbohydrate, 3 g dietary fiber, 3 g sugars, 0 g added sugars, 4 g protein, 80 mg phosphorus

Asparagus: It's Got Benefits

Most people tend to eat asparagus because it's so darn tasty—especially when it's grilled, like in this recipe. But it's okay if you just want to eat it since it's a highly nutritious food. Either way, you'll reap it's benefits as a low-calorie, fiber-packed, antioxidant-rich, non-starchy veggie.

And for people with diabetes, you're in luck again. Regularly eating asparagus may play a role in managing type 2 diabetes by helping to regulate blood glucose levels. It may help to boost insulin production in your body, too.

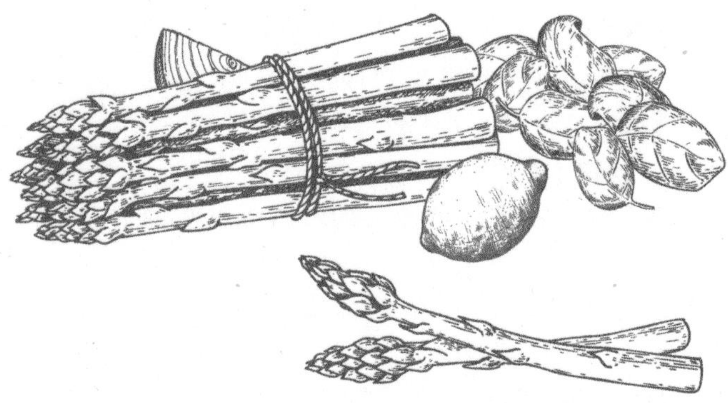

MAITAKE POWERHOUSE SALAD

A side salad doesn't have to be an afterthought. Maitake mushrooms, also called hen of the woods, makes this side salad an attention grabber. The earthy, tangy, and fresh flavors along with its textures will keep your attention. The nutritional richness of the greens (try baby spinach, organic baby kale, and/or chopped chard) will make this recipe one that should be enjoyed often.

SERVES: 4 I SERVING SIZE: 1 ½ cups salad with 1 large mushroom
PREP TIME: 12 minutes I COOK TIME: 6 to 7 minutes

- 1½ teaspoons sunflower or avocado oil
- 2 (3½-ounce) maitake mushroom heads, halved, or 4 portabella mushroom caps
- ½ teaspoon freshly ground black pepper, divided
- ⅛ teaspoon sea salt, or to taste
- 6 cups packed fresh power greens, such as baby spinach, organic baby kale, and/or chopped chard (6 ounces)
- 1 small red onion, halved, very thinly sliced
- 1½ tablespoons white balsamic or aged balsamic vinegar
- 1 tablespoon extra-virgin olive oil
- 2 tablespoons finely crumbled, plant-based blue cheese or feta-style cheese*
- 1½ tablespoons raw shelled hemp seeds (optional)

**Note: Ideally, choose vegan cheese products based on tree nuts.*

DIRECTIONS

1. Heat the sunflower oil in a large, stick-resistant skillet over medium-high heat. Add the mushrooms and sauté on all sides until cooked through and browned, about 5 to 6 minutes. Season with ¼ teaspoon of the pepper and the salt.
2. Toss the greens and onion with the vinegar and olive oil in a large bowl. Arrange the salad onto four plates. Top with the sautéed mushrooms. Sprinkle with the "cheese," remaining ¼ teaspoon pepper, and, if using, the hemp seeds.

NUTRITION INFO

Choices/Exchanges: 1½ vegetable, 1½ fat

Per serving: 100 calories, 7 g total fat, 1.5 g saturated fat, 0g trans fat, 0 mg cholesterol, 170 mg sodium, 390 mg potassium, 8 g total carbohydrate, 3 g dietary fiber, 3 g sugars, 0 g added sugars, 3 g protein, 80 mg phosphorus

Mushrooms and Diabetes

Edible mushrooms, like maitake, have potential antidiabetic properties. That's because they're packed with many naturally occurring, health-protective plant compounds, including fiber, phenolics, and alkaloids. Also, they offer prebiotics that may help boost healthfulness of the gut microbiome, which may play an important role in diabetes management.

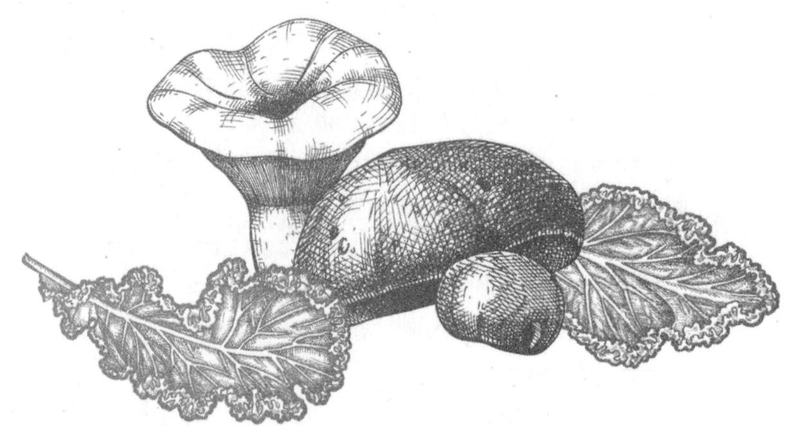

CREAMY PICNIC MACARONI SALAD

Are you planning a picnic or cookout? Then you'll definitely want to plan to make this comforting classic. Though I've given this recipe many modern twists and, of course, a vegan makeover, it still gives you all of the crave-worthy macaroni salad tastes and textures that you desire. Pick whatever noodle shape you like. And use this recipe as an opportunity to enjoy leftover roasted or grilled veggies, or fresh veggie scraps, as the non-starchy veggies of choice.

SERVES: 8 | SERVING SIZE: ¾ cup
PREP TIME: 15 minutes | COOK TIME: 10 minutes

- 8 ounces dry whole-grain reginetti, farfalle, or macaroni
- ½ cup vegan mayo or aquafaba "mayo"
- 2 tablespoons well-drained, minced pepperoncini or other pickled peppers
- 1½ tablespoons rice vinegar
- 1½ teaspoons Dijon mustard
- 1 teaspoon nutritional yeast flakes
- ½ teaspoon sea salt
- 1½ cups extra-thinly sliced, non-starchy veggies of choice, such fennel stalks and freshly roasted red bell pepper
- 2 cups packed baby arugula (2 ounces)
- 2 scallions, green and white parts, extra-thinly sliced
- ¼ teaspoon freshly ground black pepper, or to taste

DIRECTIONS

1. Cook the pasta according to package directions or per my lid-cooking technique (following recipe). Drain the pasta, toss or stir the pasta in a colander with several ice cubes (or quickly rinse under cold running water) to cool, and drain again.
2. In a large bowl, stir together the vegan mayo, pepperoncini, vinegar, mustard, nutritional yeast, and salt. Stir in the sliced veggies and cooled pasta.
3. When ready to serve, stir in the arugula and scallions. Transfer to a serving bowl, sprinkle with the black pepper, and serve.

NUTRITION INFO

Choices/Exchanges: 1½ starch, ½ vegetable, 2 fat

Per serving: 220 calories, 11 g total fat, 1 g saturated fat, 0 g trans fat, 0 mg cholesterol, 260 mg sodium, 170 mg potassium, 25 g total carbohydrate, 4 g dietary fiber, 1 g sugars, 0 g added sugars, 5 g protein, 110 mg phosphorus

Lid-Cooking Pasta

It's always a good idea to try to save energy. You can even do it while preparing pasta. Cook it using my "lid-cooking" technique: Bring the water to a boil, stir in the pasta, bring it back to a boil, cover with a lid, turn off the heat (or remove from heat if using a traditional electric stove); and let the pasta "lid-cook" (cook without heat with the lid on) undisturbed for the exact time suggested on the package, ideally using the low end of any time range given. That's it!

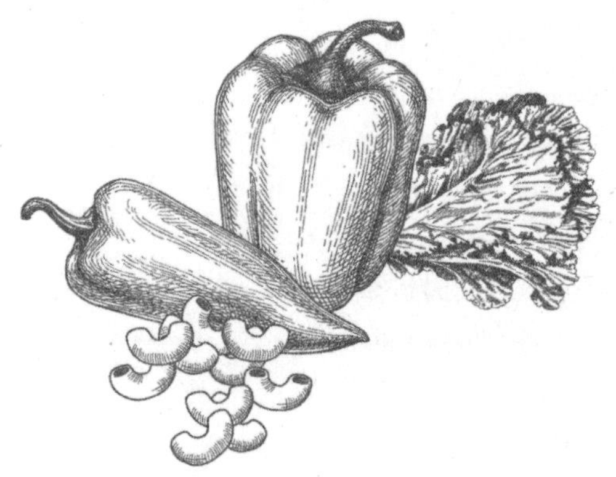

ITALIAN ROTINI AND GRILLED VEGETABLE SALAD

Being an Italian pasta salad fan for nearly my entire life, I regularly create new versions for a fresh take. But one of the challenges is that the carbs can add up quickly. I keep them in check here since this nutrient-dense pasta salad recipe is laden with grilled, non-starchy vegetables—eggplant, zucchini, onion, and fennel—which makes it intriguingly smoky and fully satisfying. The generous finish of fresh basil provides fragrant delight. There's truly taste bud excitement in every bite.

SERVES: 6 I SERVING SIZE: 1¾ cups
PREP TIME: 16 minutes I COOK TIME: 22 minutes

- 1 medium (1-pound) eggplant, unpeeled, cut into ½-inch rounds
- 1 medium (7-ounce) zucchini, unpeeled, and cut into 4 lengthwise slices
- 1 medium red onion, peeled, trimmed, and cut crosswise into 4 thick rounds (do not separate into rings)
- 1 small fennel bulb with core, stems and fronds removed, cut into 4 slices
- 3 tablespoons extra-virgin olive oil, divided
- 5 ounces whole-grain or red lentil rotini pasta
- 3 tablespoons red wine vinegar, or to taste
- 2 large garlic cloves, minced or creamed
- ⅛ teaspoon + ¾ teaspoon sea salt
- ½ teaspoon freshly ground black pepper, or to taste
- ⅓ cup thinly sliced fresh basil

DIRECTIONS

1. Prepare an outdoor or indoor grill. Lightly brush the eggplant, zucchini, onion, and fennel slices with 1 tablespoon of the oil. Grill over direct medium-high heat until fully cooked and rich grill marks form, about 5 minutes per side, turning only as needed. Set aside.
2. Cook the pasta according to package directions or per my lid-cooking technique (page 186). Drain the pasta, toss or stir the pasta in a colander with several ice cubes (or quickly rinse under cold running water) to cool, and drain again.

3. Meanwhile, whisk together the vinegar, the remaining 2 tablespoons oil, the garlic, ⅛ teaspoon of the salt, and the pepper in a large serving bowl. Add the drained pasta and toss to coat.
4. Dice the eggplant, zucchini, and onion; finely dice the fennel. Season with the remaining ¾ teaspoon salt. Stir the vegetables and basil into the pasta until just combined. Adjust seasoning, and serve.

NUTRITION INFO

Choices/Exchanges: 1½ starch, 1 vegetable, 1 fat

Per serving: 180 calories, 8 g total fat, 1 g saturated fat, 0 g trans fat, 0 mg cholesterol, 360 mg sodium, 450 mg potassium, 27 g total carbohydrate, 5 g dietary fiber, 4 g sugars, 0 g added sugars, 5 g protein, 110 mg phosphorus

Keep the Peel On

I recommend leaving the edible peel/skin on most veggies and fruits. That's because it can provide a boost of texture, color, and overall nutrition, including fiber, to a recipe. Whenever you plan to use unpeeled conventional produce in a recipe, be sure to clean and scrub it well before preparation to reduce or remove harmful pesticide residue, dirt, and grit. Scrub organic produce well, too.

SEASONAL MEDITERRANEAN FARRO SALAD

You're going to love this versatile grain salad. It's got a crave-worthy duo of sweet and salty tastes, along with lots of ingredient intrigue, especially from the farro itself. Farro is an ancient grain that's a type of wheat. It has a pleasurably chewy texture. It's secretly (or not-so-secretly now!) my favorite grain. This salad is fit for a family of four for today and tomorrow—or serve it for a party. Otherwise, if there's just one or two of you, enjoy it meal-prep style over several days. That's how I do it.

SERVES: 8 I SERVING SIZE: ¾ cup salad
PREP TIME: 10 minutes I COOK TIME: 35 minutes (plus cooling time)

- 1 cup uncooked whole (regular) farro, rinsed and drained
- 5 cups cold water
- 3 tablespoons white balsamic vinegar
- 2 tablespoons extra-virgin olive oil
- 1 cup small, bite-sized pieces fresh seasonal fruit (such as blueberries)
- 3 cups packed fresh baby arugula
- ½ teaspoon sea salt
- ½ cup shelled, roasted, salted pistachios
- ¼ cup crumbled, plant-based feta or goat-style cheese (optional)

DIRECTIONS

1. In a large saucepan, add the farro and water. Bring to a boil over high heat. Reduce heat to medium low, cover, and simmer until tender, about 30 minutes or according to package directions. Drain excess liquid from farro using a strainer.
2. In a large bowl, whisk together the vinegar and oil. Add the farro and stir. Set aside to cool for 30 minutes. Stir, then chill.
3. When the farro is cool, stir in the fruit, arugula, and salt. Sprinkle with the pistachios and, if using, plant-based cheese and serve.

NUTRITION INFO
Choices/Exchanges: 1 starch, 1 carbohydrate, 1 fat
Per serving: 190 calories, 8 g total fat, 1 g saturated fat, 0 g trans fat, 0 mg cholesterol, 150 mg sodium, 260 mg potassium, 27 g total carbohydrate, 4 g dietary fiber, 5 g sugars, 0 g added sugars, 6 g protein, 155 mg phosphorus

Can't Find Farro?

If you can't find farro at your market, use 2½ cups of another favorite cooked whole-grain in this recipe, such as bulgur, quinoa, or freekeh. Then begin with step 2 of the recipe.

Seasonal Fruit Swaps

When fruit is in season, it's at its peak of ripeness, nutritional value, color, and flavor. So go ahead and make this salad just right for the season you're in. Instead of blueberries, you can try diced fresh figs in fall, thinly sliced pear in winter, halved cherries in spring, and diced apricots in summer.

ORANGE AND HERB QUINOA SALAD

Quinoa is typically called a whole grain, but botanically it's a seed. So you'll notice that it's got a good punch of protein in it. Prepare and enjoy it as a whole grain for recipes like this. When citrus is added to quinoa, get ready to be enticed. When generously accessorized with a fresh herb "potpourri" and toasty almonds, a beautiful and satisfying salad is the result. Grow fresh mint and basil indoors to enjoy this refreshing salad all year long.

SERVES: 4 | SERVING SIZE: ¾ cup
PREP TIME: 15 minutes (plus standing and cooling time) | COOK TIME: 23 minutes

- 1 cup low-sodium vegetable broth
- ½ cup freshly squeezed orange juice with pulp or pear nectar
- ¾ cup quinoa, rinsed and drained
- Juice of ½ lemon (1½ tablespoons)
- 2 teaspoons sunflower or extra-virgin olive oil
- ¼ teaspoon + ⅛ teaspoon sea salt, or to taste
- ¼ cup chopped fresh mint leaves
- ¼ cup chopped fresh basil leaves
- 3 tablespoons sliced natural almonds, pan-toasted
- 2 teaspoons orange zest

DIRECTIONS

1. Bring the broth and orange juice to a boil in a small saucepan over high heat. Stir in the quinoa. Cover, reduce heat to low, and cook until the quinoa is nearly tender, about 20 minutes. Remove from heat and let stand covered for 5 minutes to complete the cooking process. Transfer to a large bowl. Set aside to cool for about 30 minutes, stirring occasionally to prevent sticking. Then chill in the refrigerator.
2. Meanwhile, whisk together the lemon juice, oil, and salt in a small bowl. Stir the lemon vinaigrette into the chilled quinoa until well combined. Stir in the mint and basil. Adjust seasoning.
3. Transfer the quinoa salad to individual bowls, sprinkle with the almonds and orange zest, and serve.

NUTRITION INFO
Choices/Exchanges: 1½ starch, 1 fat
Per serving: 180 calories, 6 g total fat, 0.5 g saturated fat, 0 g trans fat, 0 mg cholesterol, 260 mg sodium, 300 mg potassium, 26 g total carbohydrate, 3 g dietary fiber, 5 g sugars, 0 g added sugars, 6 g protein, 180 mg phosphorus

Mint: The Versatile Herb

While parsley, cilantro, and basil are three fresh herbs that are popularly used, mint deserves to be a star, too. In fact, it's more versatile than many people think. It can be enjoyed in both savory and sweet dishes.

Try some of my favorite uses for fresh mint (peppermint, to be precise):

1. For aromatic freshness, add fresh mint sprigs to water, sparkling water, or iced tea. Or make a brewed peppermint tea with just hot water and fresh mint--no teabag required.
2. Add more liveliness to salad by tossing some fresh mint leaves as part the greens into nearly any leafy salad.
3. For bonus antioxidants, blend a small handful of mint leaves into fruity or chocolaty smoothies.
4. For a taste twist, make a pesto with half basil and half mint--and use anywhere you normally enjoy basil pesto (and beyond), including paired with grilled vegetables or on veggie burgers.

DILL FREEKEH AND ROASTED CARROT SALAD

You've gotta love the name *"freekeh!"* And, if it's new to you, you're gonna love its complex nutty, grassy, smoky taste. Freekeh is a roasted young, green wheat grain. It has a significant amount of fiber. Lucky for everyone's health and taste buds, it's becoming more readily available. However, if you don't have freekeh, you can make this recipe with 2½ cups of any other cooked whole grain, such as bulgur wheat, brown rice, or barley. Whether made with freekeh or another grain, this recipe is designed to be served as a salad. But it's equally tasty served at room temperature or warm as a side dish, if you prefer.

SERVES: 4 I SERVING SIZE: 1 cup
PREP TIME: 18 minutes (plus chilling time) I COOK TIME: 50–52 minutes

- 1 cup dry freekeh
- ⅓ cup finely diced red onion
- 2 tablespoons extra-virgin olive oil, divided
- ¾ teaspoon sea salt, divided
- ½ teaspoon freshly ground black pepper
- 2 jumbo carrots, very thinly sliced crosswise (about ⅛ inch thick)
- Juice of ½ lemon (1½ tablespoons)
- 2 tablespoons chopped fresh dill or tarragon

DIRECTIONS

1. Cook the freekeh according to package directions. Or, add the freekeh and 3 cups cold water to a medium saucepan and bring to a boil over high heat. Stir, cover, reduce heat to low, and simmer until the freekeh is tender, about 40 minutes for whole-grain freekeh (or 20 minutes for cracked freekeh). Remove from heat and let stand for 5 minutes. Drain any remaining water. (Makes 2½ cups.)
2. Transfer the cooked freekeh to a medium bowl and immediately stir in the onion, 1 tablespoon of the oil, ½ teaspoon of the salt, and the pepper. Set aside to slightly cool, about 20 minutes, stirring a couple times. Then chill in the refrigerator.
3. Meanwhile, preheat the oven to 475°F. Add the carrots and the remaining 1 tablespoon oil to a large bowl and toss to fully coat. Add the remaining ¼ teaspoon salt and toss to fully coat. Arrange the carrots in a single layer on 2 large rimmed baking sheets and

roast until lightly caramelized, about 10–12 minutes, stirring the carrots about halfway through the cooking time.

4. Fluff the chilled freekeh with a fork. Stir in the carrots, lemon juice, and dill. Adjust seasoning and serve.

NUTRITION INFO

Choices/Exchanges: 1½ starch, 1 vegetable, 1½ fat

Per serving: 210 calories, 8 g total fat, 1 g saturated fat, 0 g trans fat, 0 mg cholesterol, 460 mg sodium, 355mg potassium, 33 g total carbohydrate, 5 g dietary fiber, 2 g sugars, 0 g added sugars, 7 g protein, 170 mg phosphorus

Should You Soak Onions?

When raw, onions can be pungent. If you like your onions on the mild side, tone down the sharpness by soaking diced or sliced onions in cold water for up to 20 minutes, then draining well and patting dry before use. However, no onion-soaking is necessary for this recipe since the raw onion is added to steamy freekeh; the heat naturally helps to tone down onion pungency.

PARTY SORGHUM SALAD WITH ARUGULA AND PISTACHIOS

This simple, yet festive grain salad is a great pick for a party as well as for those with food intolerances. It's gluten-free (as long as you use sorghum in the recipe). And it's full of culinary drama, starting with the desirably chewy sorghum—an ancient grain that's finally getting its day in the spotlight on modern tables. The peppery arugula adds freshness and liveliness to the lemony-dressed grains. Everyone is sure to love the confetti-like pop of color and texture from the pistachios and pomegranate arils, too!

SERVES: 10 | SERVING SIZE: ¾ cup salad
PREP TIME: 15 minutes | COOK TIME: 60 minutes (plus cooling time)

- 4 cups cold water
- 1 cup uncooked whole-grain sorghum, hulled barley, or farro
- Juice and zest of 1 lemon (3 tablespoons juice), divided
- 2 tablespoons extra-virgin olive oil
- 1 teaspoon sea salt, or to taste
- ¼ teaspoon freshly ground black pepper, or to taste
- 4 cups packed fresh baby arugula (4 ounces)
- ½ cup shelled, roasted, unsalted pistachios
- ⅓ cup pomegranate arils or dried tart cherries

DIRECTIONS

1. In a medium saucepan, bring the water to a boil over high heat. Add the sorghum and bring back to boil. Cover, reduce heat to medium low, and cook until tender, about 55 minutes or according to package directions. Set aside, covered, for 10 minutes to complete the cooking process.
2. In a large bowl, whisk together the lemon juice, oil, salt, and pepper. Stir in the hot sorghum. Set aside to cool for 30 minutes. Stir, then chill.
3. When the sorghum is cool, stir in the arugula, pistachios, pomegranate arils, and desired amount of lemon zest. Adjust seasoning and serve.

NUTRITION INFO

Choices/Exchanges: 1 starch, 1 fat

Per serving: 140 calories, 6 g total fat, 1 g saturated fat, 0 g trans fat, 0 mg cholesterol, 240 mg sodium, 190 mg potassium, 19 g total carbohydrate, 4 g dietary fiber, 2 g sugars, 0 g added sugars, 4 g protein, 95 mg phosphorus

What Are Pomegranate Arils?

They're fruity-fleshed pomegranate seeds. And they're rich in antioxidants, including anthocyanins. Their vibrant ruby-red color is an indicator of this.

One way to remove arils from a whole pomegranate is to cut it into four sections and rub the arils out of the peel while it's submerged in a bowl of cold water. The white, pithy part (skin) floats; the arils sink. For simplicity, recipe-ready arils ("pom-poms") may be available in your market's produce section or freezer.

TRICOLOR COLESLAW

Classic coleslaw is based on cabbage, a health-protective "superfood." A diet rich in leafy green veggies, including cabbage, is associated with a reduced risk of type 2 diabetes. Unfortunately, coleslaw can be doused with dressing, transforming that "superfood" into an overly rich side with hidden added sugar. But you can still have full, plant-based enjoyment without undesirable goopiness. This not-so-goopy dressed slaw is brightly flavored. Using tricolor slaw mix makes it brightly colored. And fruit spread provides a desirable hint of sweetness, naturally.

SERVES: 4 I SERVING SIZE: 1 cup
PREP TIME: 8 minutes I COOK TIME: 0 minutes

- 2 tablespoons fruit-sweetened apricot fruit spread (jam)*
- 2 tablespoons vegan mayo or aquafaba "mayo"*
- 2 tablespoons apple cider vinegar
- ¼ teaspoon celery salt
- 4 cups packed tricolor or other coleslaw mix (11 ounces)

***Note: Ideally, choose products without added sugars.**

DIRECTIONS

1. In a large bowl, whisk together the fruit spread, mayo, vinegar, and celery salt until well combined. Add the coleslaw mix and stir to combine.
2. Serve or store covered in the refrigerator for up to a day.

NUTRITION INFO

Choices/Exchanges: ½ fruit, 1 vegetable, 1 fat

Per serving: 90 calories, 5 g total fat, 0.8 g saturated fat, 0 g trans fat, 0 mg cholesterol, 100 mg sodium, 210 mg potassium, 10 g total carbohydrate, 2 g dietary fiber, 5 g sugars, 0 g added sugars, 0 g protein, 20 mg phosphorus

Not All Slaws Are Created Equal

One cup of "fast food" coleslaw can provide 310 calories, 21 grams of total fat, 3.5 grams of saturated fat, 410 milligrams of sodium, and 27 grams of total carbohydrates, including 21 grams of total sugars, much of which is from added sugars. Basically, it's well worth it to your health to make your own slaw . . . especially when you can do so deliciously in minutes.

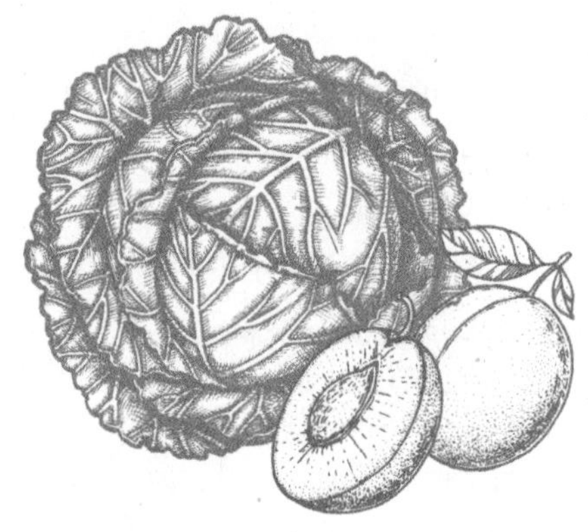

MESCLUN SALAD WITH BOSC PEARS, PECANS AND TREE-NUT CHEESE

In the fall and winter, this fancy-ish salad is one of my top picks for family, friends and, of course, myself. The perky salad is loaded with plenty of health-protective antioxidants, especially with its duo of fresh fruits. It has contrasting textures and colors that will lure you in. Though this salad will likely be most memorable due to the puréed pear dressing; it's thick, tangy, and pink.

SERVES: 4 I SERVING SIZE: 2½ cups
PREP TIME: 18 minutes I COOK TIME: 3 minutes (for toasting nuts)

- 2 medium Bosc or other pears, cored, divided
- ¼ cup apple cider vinegar
- 1½ tablespoons sunflower or flaxseed oil
- 1 medium red onion, thinly sliced, divided
- ½ teaspoon sea salt
- ¼ teaspoon ground cayenne pepper
- 8 ounces mesclun or mixed baby greens (8 cups packed)
- 1 cup seedless red grapes
- 3 tablespoons plant-based, blue cheese-style crumbles or other vegan cheese*
- 3 tablespoons chopped pecans or walnuts, pan-toasted, or roasted pistachios

**Note: Ideally, choose vegan cheese products based on tree nuts.*

DIRECTIONS

1. Chop ½ of a pear. Purée the chopped pear, vinegar, oil, ½ of the onion, salt, and cayenne pepper in a blender until smooth.
2. Just before serving, thinly slice the remaining pears. In a large bowl, toss the mesclun, grapes, sliced pears, and the remaining onion with the dressing.
3. Arrange on salad plates. Sprinkle with the cheese and pecans, and serve.

NUTRITION INFO
Choices/Exchanges: 1 fruit, 1 fat
Per serving: 150 calories, 11 g total fat, 2.5 g saturated fat, 0 g trans fat, 0 mg cholesterol, 370 mg sodium, 299 mg potassium, 13 g total carbohydrate, 5 g dietary fiber, 8 g sugars, 0 g added sugars, 2 g protein, 49 mg phosphorus

Make It Nuttier

Highlight the nutty taste by pan-toasting the pecans or walnuts just minutes before serving, sprinkling them onto each salad while still warm. Add a "layered" nut flavor by stirring in one type of nut, like walnuts, and sprinkling with a different one, like pistachios. Go for extra nuttiness by using roasted pecan, walnut, or pistachio oil in place of part or all of the sunflower or flaxseed oil. (Hint: Whichever oil you use in the recipe, consider serving the dressing on the side to give its lovely pink color the spotlight—and so everyone can add his or her desired amount.)

MESCLUN WITH BLUEBERRY VINAIGRETTE AND PLANT-BASED GOAT CHEESE

You don't need fresh blueberries to prepare this pretty salad. The frozen ones work beautifully. The leafy salad has a double dose of their vibrant purplish-blue from the blueberry vinaigrette and the whole blueberries on top. There's a creamy white contrast from the plant-based goat-style cheese and a perfect amount of crunch from the walnuts, too. It's highly nutritious thanks especially to blueberries and mesclun, which are loaded with micronutrients and antioxidants. You can make this with other fruits, too, like sliced strawberries, a medley of berries, grapes, or diced peaches.

SERVES: 4 I SERVING SIZE: 1½ cups salad
PREP TIME: 10 minutes I COOK TIME: 3 minutes (if pan-toasted walnuts)

- 1½ cups thawed frozen blueberries, divided
- 2 tablespoons white wine vinegar
- 1 tablespoon extra-virgin olive oil
- ½ teaspoon sea salt
- 1 (5-ounce) package fresh mesclun or baby spring mix
- ¼ cup chopped walnuts, pan-toasted, or roasted pistachios
- ¼ cup soft, plant-based, goat-style cheese or other soft vegan cheese*
- 2 teaspoons grated lemon zest (optional)

**Note: Ideally, choose vegan cheese products based on tree nuts.*

DIRECTIONS

1. Add ¾ cup of the blueberries, the vinegar, oil, and salt to a blender. Cover and purée for at least 1 minute on high speed.
2. Arrange the mesclun on a platter or individual plates and drizzle with the blueberry vinaigrette.
3. Top with the remaining ¾ cup blueberries, walnuts, dollops (or crumbles) of plant-based cheese and, if using, lemon zest, and serve.

NUTRITION INFO
Choices/Exchanges: 1 fruit, 2 fat
Per serving: 160 calories, 12 g total fat, 1.5 g saturated fat, 0 g trans fat, 0 mg cholesterol, 130 mg sodium, 204 mg potassium, 12 g total carbohydrate, 3 g dietary fiber, 6 g sugars, 0 g added sugars, 3 g protein, 97 mg phosphorus

Make Your Own Tree-Nut Cheese

Here's a simple way to make a plant-based cashew cheese. First, in a large jar, soak 1 cup of unroasted, unsalted cashews in 2 to 3 cups cold water in the fridge for at least 8 hours. Drain them well. Then purée (ideally in a high-powered blender) the drained cashews, 3 to 4 tablespoons cold water, 2 tablespoons lemon juice, 2 teaspoons nutritional yeast flakes, ¾ teaspoon sea salt, a pinch of onion powder, and an optional pinch of garlic powder, ground turmeric, and/or black pepper until velvety smooth. Chill and use it like soft goat cheese or cream cheese. (Makes about 1 cup; 8½ ounces.)

FRESH MINT AND BABY SPINACH SALAD WITH GRAPES

Can you smell the mint yet? So refreshing! The fresh herb is the "secret" ingredient to many of my personal salads. This one hits all of the right notes when you want a leafy salad that's fresh, fragrant, fruity, and flavorful. The salad is dressed with a fresh grape vinaigrette that's delightful. It's actually a recipe that I put together with extra ingredients I happened to have on hand one day, and it's become one of my all-time, anytime favorites.

SERVES: 4 | SERVING SIZE: 2½ cups
PREP TIME: 15 minutes | COOK TIME: 3 minutes (if pan-toasting pine nuts)

- Juice and zest of 1 small lemon (2 tablespoons juice)
- 1 tablespoon extra-virgin olive oil
- ¼ teaspoon sea salt, or to taste
- ½ teaspoon freshly ground black pepper, divided
- 1⅓ cups seedless red grapes, halved lengthwise, divided
- 5 cups packed fresh baby spinach (5 ounces)
- 2 (5-ounce) Kirby cucumbers or 10 ounces English cucumber, unpeeled, and halved lengthwise, thinly sliced crosswise
- ½ cup packed, fresh, small, whole mint leaves
- ⅓ cup extra-thinly sliced red onion
- 2 tablespoons pine nuts, pan-toasted

DIRECTIONS

1. Add the lemon juice, oil, salt, ¼ teaspoon of the pepper, and ⅓ cup of the grapes to a blender. Cover and purée. (Note: Tiny flecks from the grape skins will remain.) Set aside.
2. Toss together the spinach, cucumbers, mint, and onion in a large bowl.
3. Drizzle the grape vinaigrette over the salad and toss to coat.
4. Transfer the salad to 4 individual plates or a large platter. Sprinkle with the remaining 1 cup grapes, the pine nuts, desired amount of the lemon zest, and the remaining ¼ teaspoon pepper. Adjust seasoning and serve.

NUTRITION INFO

Choices/Exchanges: ½ fruit, 1 vegetable, 1½ fat

Per serving: 120 calories, 7 g total fat, 1 g saturated fat, 0 g trans fat, 0 mg cholesterol, 180 mg sodium, 470 mg potassium, 16 g total carbohydrate, 2 g dietary fiber, 10 g sugars, 0 g added sugars, 3 g protein, 80 mg phosphorus

Got Some Grape Ideas!

At the market, grapes are often sold in over-sized bunches in bags. If you've got a super-sized family or you're having a party, that's no problem. But what else can you do with the grapes you buy for this salad if you've got lots of extras in the fridge afterwards? Try some of my favorite grape picks.

1. Enjoy grapes as an anytime snack, ideally paired with a plant-based protein food, like pistachios.
2. Serve them as a fresh fruit swap in place of sugary jelly in a PB and J.
3. Brush grapes with olive oil, add a pinch of salt, and roast or grill (on skewers) to create intrigue in lieu of grape tomatoes, like in grain salads or guacamole.
4. Freeze them and pop into your mouth like mini frozen pops when you have a need for a bite of something sweet.
5. Whirl grapes into any fruity smoothie for an extra punch of natural sweetness.
6. Make another recipe from this cookbook that features grapes, like *Mesclun Salad with Bosc Pears, Pecans and Tree-nut Cheese* (page 199), *Tree-nut Cheese, Grape and Pistachio Poppers* (page 39) or *Grape, "Cheese" and Basil Skewers* (page 21).

Sides: Bean, Grain, and Vegetable

TUSCAN SKILLET RED BEANS

Serving this side of beans directly from the skillet makes it appealing. But once you take a bite, you'll realize it's the great taste that truly makes it a winning dish. It has distinctive Italian flavor along with so much color and texture appeal. The red beans provide a different twist since white beans are more traditional. Also consider using one or more varieties of cooked heirloom Italian beans, such as *borlotti, pavoni*, or *zolfini* beans, for bonus culinary appeal.

SERVES: 4 | serving size: ¾ cup
PREP TIME: 14 minutes | COOK TIME: 12 minutes

- 1 tablespoon extra-virgin olive oil
- 1 medium yellow onion, finely diced
- ½ cup finely diced fennel + 1 tablespoon chopped fennel fronds
- 3 cups packed, chopped, fresh organic kale leaves (3 ounces)
- 2 large garlic cloves, thinly sliced
- 1½ tablespoons red wine vinegar
- ½ teaspoon sea salt, divided
- ½ cup low-sodium vegetable broth

- 1 (15-ounce) can no-salt-added red kidney beans, drained
- 1 teaspoon grated lemon zest

DIRECTIONS

1. Heat the oil in a large, stick-resistant skillet over medium-high heat. Add the onion, the diced fennel, kale, garlic, vinegar, and ¼ teaspoon of the salt and sauté until the onion is fully softened and begins to caramelize and the kale is wilted, about 8 minutes.
2. Add the broth, beans, fennel fronds, and the remaining ¼ teaspoon salt, and sauté until the liquid is fully reduced, about 3 minutes. Adjust seasoning.
3. Sprinkle with the lemon zest, and enjoy warm served from the skillet.

NUTRITION INFO

Choices/Exchanges: 1 starch, 2 vegetable

Per serving: 140 calories, 3.5 g total fat, 0 g saturated fat, 0 g trans fat, 0 mg cholesterol, 340 mg sodium, 514 mg potassium, 20 g total carbohydrate, 10 g dietary fiber, 3 g sugars, 0 g added sugars, 8 g protein, 502 mg phosphorus

The Satiety Trio

One complaint about diabetes-friendly eating is that, for some, it may not seem satisfying. That can happen when calories are too low, or an eating plan isn't well-planned. In any case, something that can help is to try this science-backed trick. Boost satiety (the feeling of fullness) by aiming for a notable amount of this trio in every meal: protein, dietary fiber, and healthy fat. You'll get that trio here!

STEWED ROSEMARY BEAN BED

Want a side that's as comforting as mashed potatoes? These nourishing beans are so creamy they'll practically melt in your mouth. In fact, they're so scrumptious you'll want to give these beans more of a starring role on the plate. Serve them as a bed for *Vegetable Mousse "Meatloaf"* (page 117) and round out the meal with a rich-tasting, texture-filled veggie like brussels sprouts or broccoli. Or serve a well-caramelized cauliflower "roast" or "steaks" on top.

SERVES: 4 I SERVING SIZE: ½ cup
PREP TIME: 8 minutes I COOK TIME: 12 minutes

- 1 tablespoon extra-virgin olive oil
- 2 medium leeks, white and pale green parts only, halved lengthwise and thinly sliced crosswise
- Pinch of sea salt
- 1 (15-ounce) can great northern or other white beans, drained
- ¾ cup low-sodium vegetable broth
- ½ teaspoon minced fresh rosemary

DIRECTIONS

1. Heat the oil in a large saucepan over medium heat. Add the leeks and salt and cook, stirring frequently, until the leeks are softened, about 6 minutes.
2. Add the beans, broth, and rosemary and bring to a full boil over high heat. Reduce the heat to medium and simmer until the liquid is nearly evaporated, about 5 minutes, and serve.

NUTRITION INFO

Choices/Exchanges: 1½ starch, 1 vegetable, 1 fat

Per serving: 180 calories, 4 g total fat, 0.5 g saturated fat, 0 g trans fat, 0 mg cholesterol, 430 mg sodium, 454 mg potassium, 29 g total carbohydrate, 6 g dietary fiber, 4 g sugars, 0 g added sugars, 9 g protein, 160 mg phosphorus

How to Preprep Leeks

After slicing the leeks, add them to a bowl of cold water, vigorously swish them around, rinse, and drain well before using. Otherwise, they'll likely be gritty and ruin this lovely side dish.

Bean and Herb Mix and Match

You can vary the taste, texture, and look of this recipe by experimenting with different beans and herbs. Try black beans with cilantro, red kidney beans with thyme, and fava beans with mint. Be more liberal with herbs as you wish. Further kick up the flavor by adding ⅛ teaspoon dried hot pepper flakes with the broth if you like a bit

SOUTHWESTERN CILANTRO-LIME PINTOS

Trying to find a flavorful (and fast!) way to add fiber and plant protein to your meal plan? Look no further. These Southwestern-style beans provide a whopping 6 grams of dietary fiber and 8 grams of protein, which is amazing for a side dish. Of course, beans offer so much more than that, including playing a potential role in blood sugar management, reducing risk of heart disease, and providing sustained energy. And the best way to describe the culinary side of this bean dish: yum!

SERVES: 4 | SERVING SIZE: scant ½ cup
PREP TIME: 10 minutes | COOK TIME: 5 minutes

- 2 teaspoons peanut or avocado oil
- 1 large garlic clove, minced
- 1 small jalapeño pepper with some seeds, minced
- 1 (15-ounce) can pinto beans, drained
- ¼ cup low-sodium vegetable broth
- Pinch of sea salt
- ¼ cup chopped fresh cilantro
- Juice of ½ lime (1 tablespoon)

DIRECTIONS

1. Heat the oil in a medium saucepan over medium-high heat. Add the garlic and jalapeño and sauté until fragrant, about 30 seconds. Add the beans, broth, and salt and cook, stirring occasionally, until the liquid is nearly evaporated, about 3 minutes.
2. Remove from the heat and stir in the cilantro and lime juice. Serve hot as a side.

NUTRITION INFO

Choices/Exchanges: 1½ starch, ½ fat

Per serving: 140 calories, 3 g total fat, 0.5 g saturated fat, 0 g trans fat, 0 mg cholesterol, 360 mg sodium, 310 mg potassium, 22 g total carbohydrate, 6 g dietary fiber, 1 g sugars, 0 g added sugars, 8 g protein, 110 mg phosphorus

Recipe Versatility

For extra comfort, lightly top this side dish with scallion-infused, soft tree-nut cheese immediately after stirring in the cilantro and lime juice. For a more substantial side—or to transform this side into an easy entrée—stir the *Southwestern Cilantro-Lime Pintos* into cooked farro or brown rice and sprinkle with lime zest. And if you're looking for a cool side, simply chill this recipe and serve as a satisfying salad.

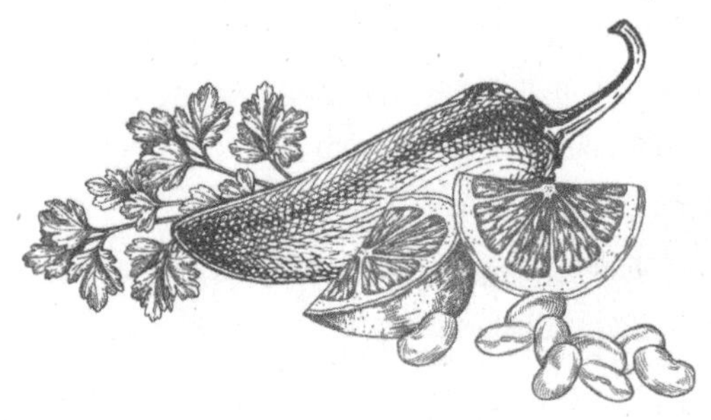

ZESTY MANDARIN EDAMAME

When dining out, edamame is often enjoyed as an appetizer eaten straight from the pod sprinkled with salt. Simple is good, but edamame is much more versatile than you might realize. When making it at home, consider going for a bit of flavor interest from time to time. Here's the way I recommend doing it: nice and spicy with a hint of orange. Not a spice fan? Simply use less hot pepper flakes.

SERVES: 4 | SERVING SIZE: ¾ cup
PREP TIME: 11 minutes | COOK TIME: 9 minutes

- 1 pound frozen, shelled, organic edamame (3½ cups)
- 2 teaspoons toasted sesame oil
- 2 teaspoons freshly grated gingerroot
- ¼ teaspoon dried hot pepper flakes
- 1½ teaspoons naturally brewed soy sauce
- 1 large garlic clove, minced
- ¼ teaspoon sea salt, or to taste
- 1½ teaspoons mandarin or navel orange zest, divided

DIRECTIONS

1. Prepare the edamame according to package directions. Drain well.
2. Heat the oil in a wok or large skillet over medium heat. Add the edamame, ginger, and hot pepper flakes, increase heat to high, and stir-fry until the edamame begins to caramelize, about 2½ minutes. Add the soy sauce, garlic, salt, and 1 teaspoon of the orange zest and stir-fry for 30 seconds. Adjust seasoning.
3. Transfer to a medium bowl or individual bowls, garnish with the remaining ½ teaspoon orange zest, and serve.

NUTRITION INFO

Choices/Exchanges: 1 starch, 2 lean protein

Per serving: 160 calories, 8 g total fat, 1 g saturated fat, 0 g trans fat, 0 mg cholesterol, 270 mg sodium, 510 mg potassium, 12 g total carbohydrate, 6 g dietary fiber, 3 g sugars, 0 g added sugars, 13 g protein, 190 mg phosphorus

Ginger Facts

Ginger isn't actually a root, it's a rhizome. When it's eaten regularly over a period of time, it imparts health benefits. These include the potential ability to help manage blood glucose or improve A1C levels for people with type 2 diabetes. Other benefits of ginger may include providing anti-inflammatory properties and gastrointestinal relief.

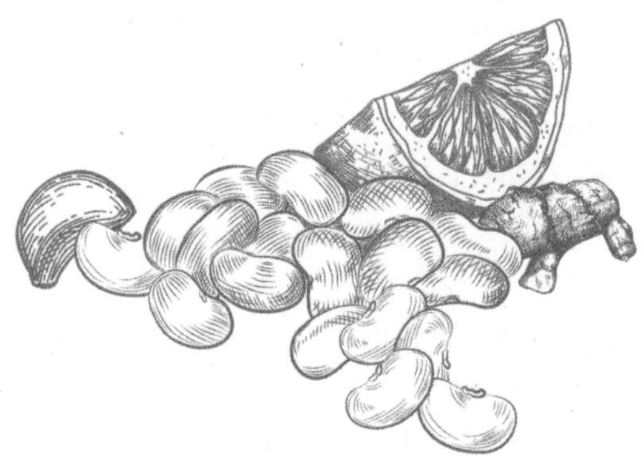

STICKY THAI QUINOA

You may have had or at least heard of sticky rice, but have you had sticky quinoa? Now is your chance. It's a foolproof recipe since the hint of mushiness is a desirable thing here. But don't prepare it just because it's sticky; make it because it's sumptuous. The culinary synergy of lemongrass, ginger, and coconut milk provide Thai flair and fragrance, while the turmeric imparts a distinguishing yellow hue. It's lovely.

SERVES: 6 | SERVING SIZE: ⅔ cup
PREP TIME: 18 minutes | COOK TIME: 37 minutes

- 1 tablespoon avocado oil or peanut oil
- 1 sweet onion, finely chopped
- 1 tablespoon freshly grated lemongrass
- Juice of ½ lime (1 tablespoon)
- ¾ teaspoon sea salt, divided
- 2 teaspoons freshly grated gingerroot
- ¼ teaspoon ground turmeric
- ⅛ teaspoon freshly ground black pepper
- 1 cup dry quinoa, rinsed and well drained
- 15 fluid ounces low-sodium vegetable broth (1⅞ cups)
- 3 tablespoons light organic coconut milk
- ¼ cup thinly sliced fresh basil + 6 sprigs basil

DIRECTIONS

1. Heat the oil in a large saucepan over medium heat. Add the onion, lemongrass, lime juice, and ¼ teaspoon of the salt and sauté until the onion is fully softened, about 8 minutes. Add the ginger, turmeric, and black pepper and sauté for 1 minute.
2. Add the quinoa, broth, and the remaining ½ teaspoon salt and bring to a boil over high heat. Cover, reduce heat to low, and cook until the quinoa is al dente and the broth is absorbed, about 20 minutes, while only partially covering during the final 5 minutes. Immediately stir in the coconut milk. Adjust seasoning.
3. Stir in the sliced basil, garnish with the basil sprigs, and serve.

NUTRITION INFO

Choices/Exchanges: 1½ starch, 1 fat

Per serving: 150 calories, 4.5 g total fat, 0.5 g saturated fat, 0 g trans fat, 0 mg cholesterol, 340 mg sodium, 240 mg potassium, 24 g total carbohydrate, 3 g dietary fiber, 5 g sugars, 0 g added sugars, 5 g protein, 150 mg phosphorus

What to Do with Extra Coconut Milk

Freeze it. I pour it into an ice cube tray—1½ tablespoons per cube—and then pop it into the freezer. Once the coconut milk cubes are frozen, I transfer them to a silicone pouch or sealable container for later use. Thaw in the fridge in a small jar overnight. You'll need 2 cubes to make this recipe again. Also, plan to use it in *Skillet Beans and Greens with Coconutty Riced Cauliflower* (page 169)—thaw 2 cubes for it—and *Caribbean Black Bean Bowl* (page 163)—thaw 6 cubes for it.

CARAMELIZED RICED CAULIFLOWER

It looks a lot like rice. And you can enjoy it just like rice. But this cauliflower side has fewer carbs and a wealth of plant nutrients. It's got plenty of flavor thanks in part to turmeric and black pepper. Plus the browning kicks up cauliflower's natural, savory sweetness. So don't get antsy and cook this recipe for just a few minutes—go for the full 10-ish minutes. Serve as is or try it in *Skillet Beans and Greens with Coconutty Riced Cauliflower.* (page 169)

SERVES: 4 I SERVING SIZE: ½ cup
PREP TIME: 8 minutes I COOK TIME: 11 minutes

- 1 pound cauliflower florets (4 cups packed)
- 2 teaspoons avocado oil or sunflower oil
- ¼ teaspoon sea salt
- ¼ teaspoon freshly ground black pepper
- ¼ teaspoon ground turmeric
- 1 to 2 tablespoons chopped fresh cilantro (optional)

DIRECTIONS

1. Add the cauliflower florets to a food processor (in batches, if necessary). Cover and pulse until it resembles rice.
2. Heat the oil in a large, deep, cast-iron or other stick-resistant skillet over medium-high heat. Add the riced cauliflower, salt, pepper, and turmeric, and cook while stirring until cooked through and lightly browned, about 10 minutes.
3. Stir in the cilantro, if using, and serve.

NUTRITION INFO

Choices/Exchanges: 1 vegetable, ½ fat

Per serving: 50 calories, 2.5 g total fat, 0.4 g saturated fat, 0 g trans fat, 0 mg cholesterol, 170 mg sodium, 340 mg potassium, 6 g total carbohydrate, 2 g dietary fiber, 2 g sugars, 0 g added sugars, 2 g protein, 50 mg phosphorus

Turmeric Plus Pepper

Turmeric gives this cauliflower side dish a rich, golden-yellow color. That's actually an indicator of curcumin, which may have an antidiabetic effect. Black pepper contains a phenolic compound called piperine. Research suggests that if you enjoy turmeric along with black pepper, your ability to absorb turmeric's curcumin may be 2,000 percent greater thanks to pepper's piperine!

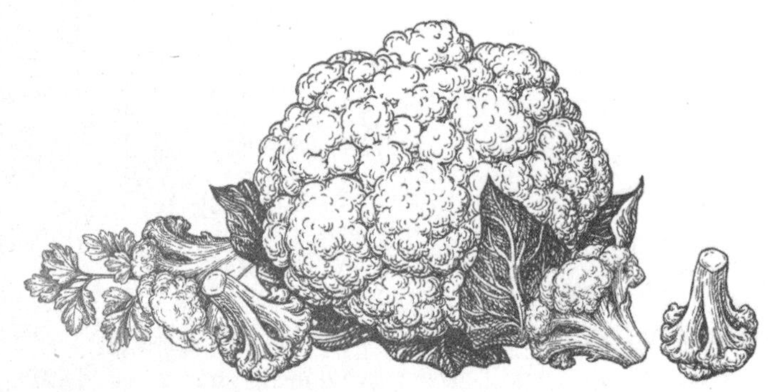

PETITE PEAS WITH PEPPERMINT

As a child, I wouldn't go near peas. Today, I find them crave-worthy. Much of their appeal has to do with preparation. This tasty, simple recipe is sure to put peas in your good graces as they're laced with a just-right amount of vegan buttery goodness. The hint of fresh mint makes them a palate-pleasing accompaniment to many Middle Eastern, Thai, and French entrées. And the cooking time of 5 minutes is just right for frozen petite peas. Dare I say it? "Easy-peasy!" Serve these sweet peas as is or toss with brown rice or a whole-grain of your choice to create an extra-enticing side.

SERVES: 4 I SERVING SIZE: scant ½ cup
PREP TIME: 5 minutes I COOK TIME: 5 minutes

- 1 (10-ounce) package frozen petite or baby peas
- 2 tablespoons unsweetened peppermint tea or water
- 2 teaspoons vegan butter
- ½ teaspoon sea salt
- 2 teaspoons finely chopped fresh mint (peppermint)

DIRECTIONS

1. Add the peas, tea, vegan butter, and salt to a medium saucepan and cook over medium heat, stirring constantly, until hot, about 5 minutes.
2. Stir in the mint and serve.

NUTRITION INFO

Choices/Exchanges: ½ starch, ½ fat

Per serving: 70 calories, 2 g total fat, 1.5 g saturated fat, 0 g trans fat, 0 mg cholesterol, 380 mg sodium, 111 mg potassium, 10 g total carbohydrate, 3 g dietary fiber, 4 g sugars, 0 g added sugars, 4 g protein, 60 mg phosphorus

Which Mint to Pick

At a farmer's market, you might have a choice between fresh peppermint and spearmint. Pick the peppermint—it's more pungent. Or, for a change of taste, try fresh tarragon instead of mint in this recipe. (Personally speaking, tarragon is an underrated herb.)

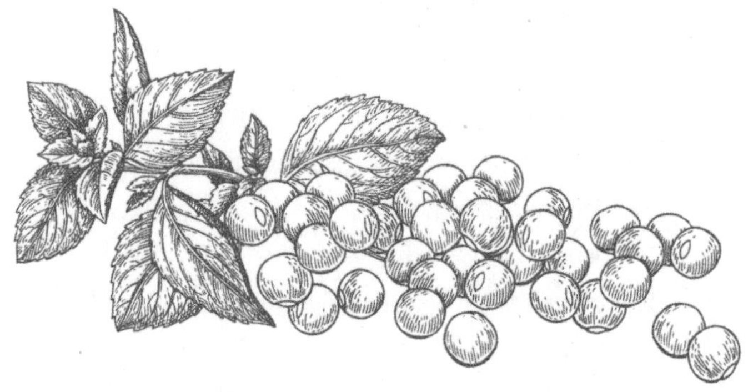

ROASTED GREEK EGGPLANT WITH PLANT-BASED FETA

I can't tell you how many times I wanted to stomp into a restaurant kitchen and tell them that no matter how delicious my entrée might have been, my side dish was second-rate, at best. Sides shouldn't be thought of as afterthoughts. They deserve as much culinary love and attention as the main dish, even for home cooks. If you're looking for a wow-worthy side dish, this roasted eggplant recipe is it. The finishing touches of fresh herbs, plant-based feta, and lemon zest make this side more like the star of the plate.

SERVES: 4 I SERVING SIZE: 2 wedges
PREP TIME: 12 minutes I COOK TIME: 30 minutes

- 3 tablespoons no-sugar-added marinara sauce of choice
- Juice and zest of ½ small lemon (1 tablespoon juice), divided
- 1 tablespoon extra-virgin olive oil
- 1 large garlic clove, minced
- ¼ teaspoon sea salt
- ¼ teaspoon ground cinnamon
- 2 small (14-ounce) eggplants, each quartered lengthwise, stems removed
- 3 tablespoons chopped, fresh, flat-leaf parsley
- 1 tablespoon chopped fresh mint or 1 teaspoon chopped fresh oregano
- 3 tablespoons finely crumbled plant-based feta cheese*

**Note: Ideally, choose vegan cheese products based on tree nuts.*

DIRECTIONS

1. Preheat the oven to 400°F. In a small bowl, whisk together the marinara sauce, lemon juice, oil, garlic, salt, and cinnamon. Arrange the eggplant wedges, skin side down, on a baking sheet lined with a silicone baking mat, or unbleached parchment paper-lined baking sheet. Generously brush the cut surfaces of the eggplant wedges with the marinara mixture.
2. Roast the eggplant wedges until fully cooked, about 30 minutes.
3. Transfer to a platter, sprinkle with the parsley, mint, plant-based feta, and lemon zest, and serve. (Hint: For an extra-luscious appearance, consider spritzing the roasted eggplant with organic olive oil cooking spray before garnishing.)

NUTRITION INFO
Choices/Exchanges: 2½ vegetable, 1 fat
Per serving: 110 calories, 6 g total fat, 2.5 g saturated fat, 0 g trans fat, 0 mg cholesterol, 250 mg sodium, 471 mg potassium, 13 g total carbohydrate, 5 g dietary fiber, 6 g sugars, 0 g added sugars, 2 g protein, 50 mg phosphorus

Salt, Pepper, and Cinnamon

Stash cinnamon next to your salt and pepper shakers. You can use cinnamon to add flavor and a touch of intriguing sweetness to both savory and sweet dishes instead of adding more salt or sugar. Try it.

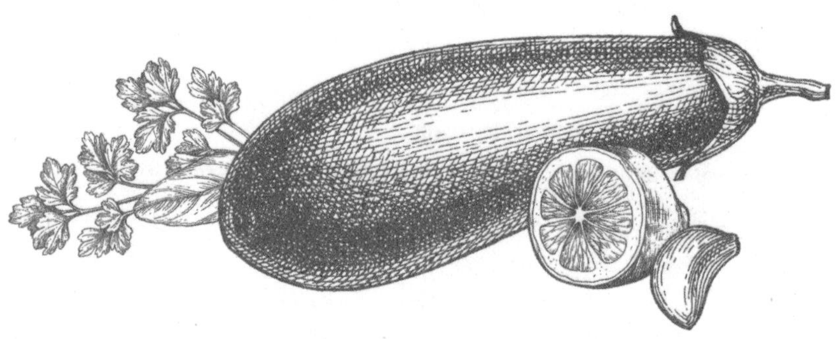

TAHINI-DRESSED ROASTED EGGPLANT ROUNDS WITH POMEGRANATE AND MINT

Do you like Middle Eastern cuisine? You'll love this dazzling side dish of tahini-dressed roasted eggplant rounds, arranged in layers that are lovingly interspersed with fresh mint. The tahini sauce adds such rich, comforting appeal in a nutritious way. The pomegranate arils provide a pop of color—and health-promoting antioxidants. This dish is a showstopper as a side, so also consider serving it as a stand-alone appetizer.

SERVES: 4 | SERVING SIZE: 3 eggplant rounds
PREP TIME: 15 minutes | COOK TIME: 30 minutes

- 1 large (1¼-pound) eggplant, cut crosswise into 12 slices
- 1½ tablespoons extra-virgin olive oil, divided
- ¼ teaspoon + ⅛ teaspoon sea salt, or to taste
- 3 tablespoons tahini
- 3 tablespoons unsweetened green or peppermint tea
- Juice of 1 small lemon (2 tablespoons)
- 1 large garlic clove, minced
- Pinch of ground cumin, or to taste
- 16 large, fresh, flat-leaf mint leaves + 4 sprigs
- ¼ cup pomegranate arils

DIRECTIONS

1. Preheat the oven to 450°F. Lightly brush both sides of the eggplant slices with 1 tablespoon of the olive oil. Sprinkle with ¼ teaspoon of the salt. Arrange onto a large silicone baking mat, or unbleached, parchment-paper-lined baking sheet. Roast in the oven until fully cooked and lightly browned, about 30 minutes, flipping over eggplant rounds about halfway through the roasting process.
2. Meanwhile, whisk together until smooth the tahini, tea, lemon juice, garlic, cumin, and the remaining ½ tablespoon olive oil and ⅛ teaspoon salt in a medium bowl or liquid measuring cup. Adjust seasoning.
3. Onto plates or a platter, arrange 4 stacks of 3 eggplant rounds each, placing the largest round on the bottom of each stack. Alternatively, fan out the eggplant rounds on a plate rather than stacking them. Position the mint leaves between the layers, allowing the

leaves to peek out. Drizzle each stack with about 2 tablespoons of the tahini dressing and 1 tablespoon of the pomegranate arils. Then garnish with the mint sprigs and serve warm.

NUTRITION INFO

Choices/Exchanges: 2 vegetable, 1 fat

Per serving: 100 calories, 6 g total fat, 1 g saturated fat, 0 g trans fat, 0 mg cholesterol, 230 mg sodium, 406 mg potassium, 12 g total carbohydrate, 6 g dietary fiber, 7 g sugars, 0 g added sugars, 2 g protein, 47 mg phosphorus

Vintage Cuisine

What do you call a dish that you make with leftovers? I call it "vintage cuisine"! You can make your own here if you have any leftovers. Add the eggplant and tahini dressing (without the pomegranate arils) to a food processor and purée with an extra splash of lemon juice to make a delicious roasted eggplant dip. There's no need to remove the eggplant peel (unless you want to)—it adds cuisine interest and nutrition.

ROSEMARY ROASTED ROOT VEGETABLES

Roasting veggies is a wonderful way to enjoy all of their bountiful benefits, especially in the fall and winter. And choosing a variety of roots, like parsnips and turnips, as well as tubers, like sweet potatoes, is one way to assure you're getting a variety of beneficial nutrients. But perhaps the best part of this recipe is the scent of rosemary that will waft through your home during roasting, making these vegetables even more enticing.

SERVES: 6 I SERVING SIZE: ⅔ cup
PREP TIME: 15 minutes I COOK TIME: 1 hour

- 2 large parsnips, peeled and sliced crosswise into ¾-inch-thick coins
- 1 large turnip, peeled and sliced crosswise into 1-inch-thick pieces, then into wedges
- 1 medium sweet potato, peeled or unpeeled, sliced crosswise into 1-inch-thick pieces, then into half rounds
- 1½ tablespoons extra-virgin olive oil, divided
- 2 teaspoons finely chopped fresh rosemary
- ¾ teaspoon sea salt
- 1 large leek, white and pale green parts only, halved lengthwise and sliced crosswise into 1-inch-thick half rounds
- 4 large garlic cloves, minced

DIRECTIONS

1. Preheat the oven to 400°F. Add the parsnips, turnip, sweet potato, 1 tablespoon of the oil, the rosemary, and salt to a large bowl and toss to coat.
2. Transfer the vegetables to a baking sheet lined with a silicone baking mat, or unbleached, parchment-paper-lined, large, rimmed baking sheet and roast for 20 minutes. Stir in the leeks and roast for 20 minutes more.
3. In a small bowl, combine the garlic with the remaining ½ tablespoon oil. Stir the garlic mixture into the roasted vegetables and roast until the vegetables are tender and lightly browned, about 20 minutes more. Then serve.

NUTRITION INFO

Choices/Exchanges: ½ starch, 3 vegetable, ½ fat

Per serving: 130 calories, 3.5 g total fat, 0.5 g saturated fat, 0 g trans fat, 0 mg cholesterol, 350 mg sodium, 455 mg potassium, 24 g total carbohydrate, 5 g dietary fiber, 6 g sugars, 0 g added sugars, 2 g protein, 80 mg phosphorus

Time and Taste Twists

You can roast these veggies in advance and then place into a 450°F oven to reheat for about 10 minutes. This way you'll be able to perfectly time them to serve along with your entrée. You can also periodically swap out one of the vegetables for carrots, celery root (celeriac), or beets. It's an enticing way to experience new veggies, too.

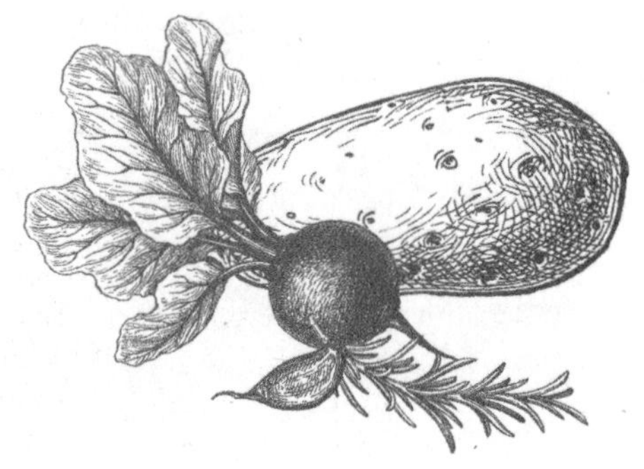

SPRING ASPARAGUS STIR-FRY

When asparagus is at its peak in spring, this side is so appetizing. Try white or purple asparagus, not just the usual green variety, when you can find them. Whichever color you choose, you'll find that stir-fries like this are ideal for side dishes, not just main dishes. Try pairing this simple, sweet-n-salty asparagus stir-fry with *Blackened Orange and Ginger Tofu Filets* (page 119) and brown basmati rice. It's oh so good—and good for you.

SERVES: 4 | SERVING SIZE: 1 rounded cup
PREP TIME: 10 minutes | COOK TIME: 7 minutes

- 2 tablespoons naturally brewed reduced-sodium soy sauce
- 1 tablespoon coconut nectar or date syrup
- 2 teaspoons toasted sesame oil
- 2 large garlic cloves, minced
- 1 teaspoon grated fresh gingerroot
- 2 pounds asparagus, ends trimmed, cut on diagonal into 2-inch-long pieces
- ⅛ teaspoon sea salt
- 1 teaspoon sesame seeds, roasted or pan-toasted

DIRECTIONS

1. Stir together the soy sauce and coconut nectar in a small bowl and set aside.
2. Heat the oil in a large skillet or wok over medium-high heat. (Reduce the heat if the oil begins to smoke.) Add the garlic and ginger and sauté until fragrant, about 30 seconds.
3. Add the thick-stemmed asparagus pieces and stir-fry for 1 minute. Add the thin-stemmed asparagus pieces and stir-fry for 1 minute. Add the asparagus tips and stir-fry until tender-crisp, about 2 minutes.
4. Add the soy sauce-coconut nectar mixture and cook while tossing to fully coat the asparagus, about 1 minute. Sprinkle with salt. Transfer the asparagus with any remaining sauce to a serving bowl, sprinkle with the sesame seeds, and serve.

NUTRITION INFO

Choices/Exchanges: 1½ vegetable, ½ fat

Per serving: 70 calories, 2.5 g total fat, 0 g saturated fat, 0 g trans fat, 0 mg cholesterol, 370 mg sodium, 314 mg potassium, 11 g total carbohydrate, 3 g dietary fiber, 6 g sugars, 4 g added sugars, 4 g protein, 78 mg phosphorus

Skinny Is In . . . for Asparagus

The skinnier, the speedier when it comes to asparagus cookery. So if you can find them, choose pencil-like asparagus spears. Without thick stems, little trimming is required. And the pieces can be stir-fried all at once—for about 2 to 2½ minutes total.

Do You Need a Wok for Stir-Frying?

The short answer is "no." Like in this recipe, stir-frying can be done in a skillet, such as a well-seasoned cast-iron skillet. And one that's large enough so that the food you're stir-frying, like asparagus, actually gets stir-fried and not steamed. However, if you have or can get a wok, I highly recommend it. If you cook on a gas range, a traditional carbon steel wok heats up quickly, distributes heat well, and allows you to "push" cooked food up the sides while the lesser-cooked food remains in the hottest center. If you have an induction or flat electric cooktop, be sure to choose a wok that's flat-bottomed.

WOK-SAUTÉED BRUSSELS SPROUTS

Brussels sprouts have been a long-celebrated vegetable at Thanksgiving tables in America. Luckily for everyone's health, these cute little cabbages have been popping up at family mealtimes, friend gatherings, and quaint couple and solo dinners all year long. When prepared right, they're a true savory delight. You'll find this Chinese-inspired preparation a unique and delicious way to enjoy this veggie any day.

SERVES: 4 | SERVING SIZE: ¾ cup
PREP TIME: 12 minutes | COOK TIME: 15 minutes

- 1¼ cups low-sodium vegetable broth
- 1½ teaspoons rice or brown rice vinegar
- 1 pound trimmed brussels sprouts, quartered lengthwise
- 1 small or ½ large red onion, finely diced
- 1 tablespoon + 1 teaspoon avocado oil or sunflower oil
- ½ teaspoon sea salt, or to taste
- ¼ teaspoon freshly ground black pepper, or to taste
- 1 teaspoon naturally brewed soy sauce
- 1½ tablespoons chopped fresh cilantro, or to taste

DIRECTIONS

1. Bring the broth and vinegar to a boil in a wok or extra-large skillet over medium-high heat. Add the brussels sprouts and onion and cook while stirring until no liquid remains, about 8 minutes. Add the oil, salt, and pepper and sauté until the sprouts are crisp-tender and caramelized, about 4 minutes. Sprinkle with the soy sauce and cilantro and toss to coat. Adjust seasoning.
2. Transfer to individual bowls or a large serving bowl and serve.

NUTRITION INFO
Choices/Exchanges: 2 vegetable, 1 fat
Per serving: 100 calories, 5 g total fat, 0 g saturated fat, 0 g trans fat, 0 mg cholesterol, 440 mg sodium, 420 mg potassium, 12 g total carbohydrate, 4 g dietary fiber, 4 g sugars, 0 g added sugars, 4 g protein, 70 mg phosphorus

Brussels Sprouts and Diabetes

Eating cruciferous vegetables, like brussels sprouts, can play a role in improving overall health and reducing the risk of diabetes, among other chronic medical conditions. Brussels sprouts contain sulforaphane, which is a plant nutrient that offers anti-inflammatory properties. Chronic inflammation is associated with type 2 diabetes, heart disease, and beyond. That means eating foods containing anti-inflammatory nutrients, like you find in brussels sprouts, may help to reduce inflammation in your body and, therefore, be beneficial in the management of type 2 diabetes.

EASY MIDDLE-EASTERN GREEN BEANS

The short name for a Lebanese dish that I grew up on is *loubieh.* It's a fragrant, comforting, stewy green bean and tomato dish. My mom usually made it with cubes of beef as well, though my preference is going beef free! While this easy recipe is not loubieh, it's my simplified, loose interpretation of it. It's just green beans and grape tomatoes cooked with a just-right amount of extra-virgin olive oil and seasoned with cinnamon and sea salt. I hope it makes you smile as much as it does me.

SERVES: 2 | SERVING SIZE: about 1½ cups
PREP TIME: 6 minutes | COOK TIME: 11 to 13 minutes

- 1 tablespoon extra-virgin olive oil
- 8 ounces fresh green beans, stem ends trimmed
- 1 cup grape tomatoes (6 ounces)
- ¼ teaspoon ground cinnamon, or to taste
- ⅛ teaspoon sea salt, or to taste

DIRECTIONS

1. Heat the oil in a large, cast-iron or other stick-resistant skillet over medium heat. Add the green beans and tomatoes, cover, and cook until the green beans are crisp-tender and tomatoes are fully softened, about 10 to 12 minutes, tossing with tongs or shaking the skillet a couple times throughout the cooking.
2. Sprinkle with the cinnamon and salt and toss to combine. Adjust seasoning and serve.

NUTRITION INFO

Choices/Exchanges: 2 vegetable, 1½ fat

Per serving: 110 calories, 7 g total fat, 1 g saturated fat, 0 g trans fat, 0 mg cholesterol, 150 mg sodium, 365 mg potassium, 12 g total carbohydrate, 5 g dietary fiber, 6 g sugars, 0 g added sugars, 3 g protein, 53 mg phosphorus

Recipe Extras

I enjoy this recipe's simplicity. But absolutely add your own special touch, if you like. For a nutty accent, sprinkle with pan-toasted pine nuts or sliced almonds. For a generous side, combine with steamed whole grains, like farro, freekeh, or brown rice, then squirt with lemon. For extra pops of color, use a colorful variety of grape tomatoes. Or for a Mexican-style interpretation, sprinkle with cumin and chili powder instead of cinnamon.

GRAPE TOMATO SUCCOTASH

Practically every time I hear the word succotash, I want to shout the Sylvester the Cat phrase, "Sufferin' succotash!" So funny. But this dish is whatever the opposite of "sufferin'" is. Though succotash is usually associated with summertime cuisine when corn is in season, this wholesome recipe is designed to be enjoyed anytime you're able to pick up a pint of grape tomatoes. And since you can use frozen corn and lima beans here, you can savor this veggie dish often. It's as colorful as it is flavorful.

SERVES: 4 | SERVING SIZE: 1 rounded cup
PREP TIME: 15 minutes | COOK TIME: 11 minutes

- 1 tablespoon extra-virgin olive oil
- 1 medium red onion, diced
- 1 pound fresh lima beans in pods, shelled, or 10 ounces thawed frozen lima beans (2 cups)
- 1 cup fresh (from 2 medium ears) or thawed frozen yellow sweet corn
- ½ small jalapeño pepper, with seeds, thinly sliced crosswise
- ¾ cup unsweetened, plant-based milk of choice (I like sunflower milk here)
- ½ teaspoon + ⅛ teaspoon sea salt
- 1 pint grape tomatoes, quartered lengthwise
- 1 tablespoon apple cider vinegar
- 3 tablespoons finely chopped fresh cilantro, or to taste

DIRECTIONS

1. Heat the oil in a large skillet over medium-high heat. Add the onion, lima beans, corn, and jalapeño, and sauté until the vegetables are heated through, about 3 minutes. Add the plant-based milk and salt, and sauté until the vegetables are tender and liquid is fully reduced, about 6 minutes. Add the tomatoes and vinegar and sauté until the tomatoes are heated through, about 1 minute. Stir in the cilantro. Adjust seasoning.
2. Transfer to a serving bowl or individual bowls, garnish with additional cilantro, if desired, and serve.

NUTRITION INFO
Choices/Exchanges: 2 starch, 1 fat
Per serving: 200 calories, 4.5 g total fat, 0.5 g saturated fat, 0 g trans fat, 0 mg cholesterol, 440 mg sodium, 694 mg potassium, 33 g total carbohydrate, 7 g dietary fiber, 5 g sugars, 0 g added sugars, 8 g protein, 141 mg phosphorus

Corn Benefits

Sometimes corn gets a bad rap. But you may be pleasantly surprised to know that it counts as a whole grain. Corn is a good source of vitamin C, which acts as an antioxidant to protect your body's cells. And it's a notable source of lutein and zeaxanthin, which are carotenoids that may help protect eye health.

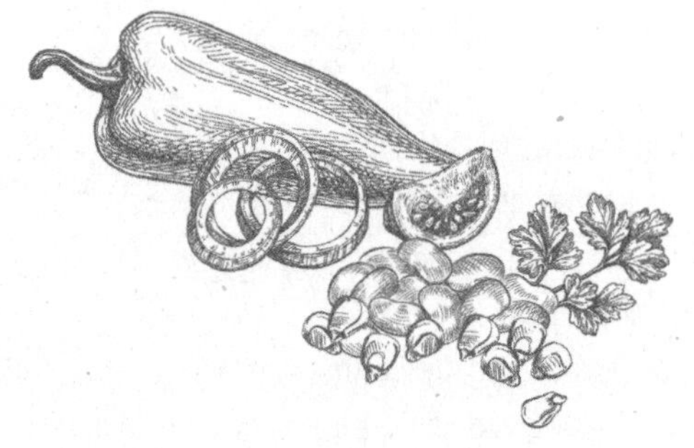

GARLIC SAUTEÉED RAPINI WITH TART CHERRIES

It's not broccoli, it's broccoli raab. Or call it by its sassier name, rapini. Either way, it's a taste-bud thriller in this sweet, salty, and bitter preparation, with a hint of heat. It's sure to please anyone into big taste. The rapini's noteworthy bitterness is beautifully balanced in this side dish recipe with pleasant pops of cherries. Get ready to be wowed.

SERVES: 4 | SERVING SIZE: about 1 cup
PREP TIME: 12 minutes | COOK TIME: 35 minutes

- 1 whole, small garlic bulb
- 1 tablespoon extra-virgin olive oil, divided
- ½ cup low-sodium vegetable broth
- 3 tablespoons dried tart cherries
- 1 (1-pound) bunch rapini (broccoli raab), stems trimmed
- ¼ teaspoon sea salt, or to taste
- ¼ teaspoon freshly ground black pepper, or to taste
- ¼ teaspoon dried hot pepper flakes
- 1 tablespoon red wine vinegar

DIRECTIONS

1. Cut the top portion off of the garlic to expose all the cloves. Rub with ½ teaspoon of the oil. Wrap in recycled aluminum foil. Bake in a toaster oven (or preheated conventional oven) at 375°F until fully softened, about 25 minutes. When cool enough to handle, squeeze the softened garlic cloves from the skins. Fully smash the cloves.
2. Bring the broth, cherries, and garlic to a boil in a large, deep skillet over medium-high heat. Add the rapini and cook while tossing until no liquid remains, about 3 minutes.
3. Add the remaining 2½ teaspoons oil, salt, black pepper, and hot pepper flakes and toss with tongs until the rapini is crisp-tender, about 3 minutes. Toss with the vinegar. Adjust seasoning.
4. Transfer the rapini to individual plates or a platter, and serve.

NUTRITION INFO

Choices/Exchanges: ½ fruit, 1 vegetable, 1 fat

Per serving: 90 calories, 4 g total fat, 0.5 g saturated fat, 0 g trans fat, 0 mg cholesterol, 200 mg sodium, 280 mg potassium, 11 g total carbohydrate, 3 g dietary fiber, 5 g sugars, 2 g added sugars, 4 g protein, 90 mg phosphorus

The Acid Trick

Examples of a culinary acids include lemon juice, lime juice, and vinegars. In this recipe, you'll notice red wine vinegar as the acid of choice. In cuisine, using it can help to balance a bitter taste found in certain vegetables, such as rapini. So if you think a vegetable-based preparation seems too bitter, consider adding a little acid to it.

I like to somewhat match the acid of choice to the food, kind of like wine pairing. But it's ultimately best to choose what you like best. For instead, add a squirt of lemon to spinach dishes or Middle Eastern plant-based dishes in general. Balance Mexican vegan dishes, like mushroom tacos, with a squirt of lime. Drizzle balsamic or red wine vinegar into Italian tomato-based dishes. And if you've got a cup or bowl of soup that needs more taste balance, finish it with a little splash of cider vinegar.

SAUTÉED BABY SPINACH WITH CURRANTS AND PINE NUTS

Spinach is one of the most popular vegetables in America. But at restaurants, too often a side of spinach is served either plain and steamed or overly rich and creamed. Here's how do it better. You—and anyone you serve this to—will enjoy this slightly fruity, slightly nutty version of sautéed baby spinach. And at only 80 calories a serving (if you're counting), you can (and should!) enjoy it often.

SERVES: 4 | SERVING SIZE: ½ cup
PREP TIME: 8 minutes | COOK TIME: 8 minutes

- 2 teaspoons extra-virgin olive oil
- 1 large garlic clove, thinly sliced
- 1 pound fresh baby spinach
- Juice of ½ lemon (1½ tablespoons) plus 4 lemon wedges, divided
- 1 tablespoon currants or chopped dried tart cherries
- ¼ teaspoon sea salt
- ⅛ teaspoon dried hot pepper flakes, or to taste
- 1½ tablespoons pine nuts, pan-toasted

DIRECTIONS

1. Heat the oil in an extra-large skillet over medium heat. Add the garlic and sauté until it just begins to lightly brown, about 2 minutes. Transfer the garlic to a small dish and set aside.
2. Add the spinach to the skillet one large handful at a time. Cook and toss with tongs until all the spinach is just wilted, about 4 minutes. Add the lemon juice and currants and toss to combine, about 30 seconds. Remove from heat and sprinkle with the salt and hot pepper flakes.
3. Using tongs, transfer the spinach to a serving bowl or platter. Top with the reserved garlic slices and the pine nuts, and serve with the lemon wedges.

NUTRITION INFO

Choices/Exchanges: 1½ vegetable, 1 fat

Per serving: 80 calories, 5 g total fat, 0.5 g saturated fat, 0 g trans fat, 0 mg cholesterol, 240 mg sodium, 689 mg potassium, 8 g total carbohydrate, 3 g dietary fiber, 2 g sugars, 0 g added sugars, 4 g protein, 79 mg phosphorus

Spinach Is a Superfood

One of the key nutrients in spinach is lutein, an antioxidant that may reduce the risk of age-related macular degeneration—the leading cause of blindness in older adults. And there's more good news for spinach lovers. One study found that folks with the highest versus the lowest magnesium intake were about half as likely to get type 2 diabetes. Guess what's rich in magnesium? Spinach! Almonds, beans, and avocados are excellent sources of this mineral, too.

CITRUS BRAISED KALE

Kale is a trendy green, which is awesome. It's super nutrient rich and packs a punch of delightful yet slightly bitter tones. In this recipe, its taste is totally balanced by the fresh sweetness from the orange, richness from the hint of vegan butter, and "heat" from the hot pepper flakes. To top that, it's simple to prepare. You'll want to make this kale recipe a go-to side often.

SERVES: 4 | SERVING SIZE: 1¼ cups
PREP TIME: 8 minutes | COOK TIME: 11 minutes

- 2 teaspoons vegan butter or extra-virgin olive oil
- 1 pound chopped fresh organic kale
- ¼ cup freshly squeezed orange juice with pulp + 1 teaspoon orange zest
- ¼ teaspoon + ⅛ teaspoon sea salt, or to taste
- ¼ teaspoon freshly ground black pepper, or to taste
- ⅛ teaspoon dried hot pepper flakes, or to taste

DIRECTIONS

1. Melt the vegan butter in a Dutch oven or extra-large deep skillet over medium-high heat. Add the kale and sauté by tossing with tongs until just wilted, about 5 minutes.
2. Add the orange juice with pulp, salt, black pepper, and hot pepper flakes and toss to combine. Cover, reduce heat to medium-low, and cook until fully softened, about 5 minutes, stirring once during braising. Adjust seasoning.
3. Sprinkle with the orange zest, and serve.

NUTRITION INFO

Choices/Exchanges: 2 vegetable, ½ fat

Per serving: 80 calories, 3 g total fat, 1.5 g saturated fat, 0 g trans fat, 0 mg cholesterol, 280 mg sodium, 588 mg potassium, 12 g total carbohydrate, 4 g dietary fiber, 4 g sugars, 0 g added sugars, 5 g protein, 107 mg phosphorus

Kale Chips

One of the coolest ways to serve kale is as chips. They're so easy to make, too. Here's what I do—no formal recipe required. Remove the stems and tough ribs from a bunch of kale (reserve for other use!) and tear up the leaves into large, bite-sized pieces. Lightly toss the leaves with a little extra-virgin olive oil, a pinch of sea salt, and any other spice you might want (I enjoy Chinese five-spice powder). Arrange in a single layer on rimmed baking sheets. And bake in a 300°F oven until crisped, about 20 minutes. Munch on them as an anytime snack.

WHIPPED PURPLE CAULIFLOWER WITH CHIVES

While you'll start with purple cauliflower, you'll wind up with midnight blue-hued cauliflower after steaming it in this recipe. It's quite dramatic . . . in a good way! Ultimately, this comforting side is a carb-friendlier and more intriguing option in place of mashed potatoes. Need an extra special touch for a special occasion? Instead of chives, drizzle the whipped purple cauliflower with a pesto sauce, like *Plant-Based Pesto.* (page 240)

SERVES: 4 | SERVING SIZE: ½ rounded cup
PREP TIME: 8 minutes | COOK TIME: 33 minutes

- 22 ounces purple cauliflower florets (from 1 large head)
- 1½ cups plain, unsweetened, plant-based milk of choice
- 2 large garlic cloves, peeled and halved
- 1 tablespoon vegan butter or extra-virgin olive oil, divided
- ½ teaspoon sea salt
- 2 teaspoons chopped fresh chives

DIRECTIONS

1. Add the purple cauliflower florets, plant-based milk, and garlic halves to a large saucepan. (Note: The plant-based milk will not completely cover the cauliflower.) Bring just to a boil over high heat. Cover tightly, reduce heat to low, and steam until the cauliflower is mashable, about 30 minutes.
2. Drain the cauliflower and garlic well through a colander, reserving the plant-based milk ("purple milk") for other use.
3. Add the cauliflower, garlic, vegan butter, and salt to a food processor or blender and purée until creamy and fluffy.
4. Transfer the whipped cauliflower to a serving bowl, sprinkle with the chives, and serve.

NUTRITION INFO
Choices/Exchanges: 2 vegetable, ½ fat
Per serving: 70 calories, 3.5 g total fat, 2.5 g saturated fat, 0 g trans fat, 0 mg cholesterol, 380 mg sodium, 496 mg potassium, 8 g total carbohydrate, 3 g dietary fiber, 3 g sugars, 0 g added sugars, 3 g protein, 74 mg phosphorus

"Purple Milk" Tips

You'll have leftover plant-based milk after steaming the cauliflower in it. Save it! You can use this midnight blue-hued "purple milk" instead of low-sodium vegetable broth or regular plant-based milk as a nourishing, flavorful addition to soups, stews, sauces, and casserole-style dishes, when a rich color or cauliflower flavor is a bonus.

Plant-Based Pesto

I don't have one recipe for pesto, I have a gazillion! Or, at least a dozen. But here's the version I like to do the most often. Hope you try it! Purée the following in a blender: 2 cups packed fresh basil leaves; ¾ cup mixture toasted/roasted nuts and seeds (like pine nuts, pistachios and hemp seeds), 2 large garlic cloves, 2 tablespoons lemon juice, 2 teaspoons nutritional yeast flakes, ½ cup extra-virgin olive oil, and sea salt and smoked paprika to taste.

Soups and Stews

COOL AVOCADO SOUP

Too hot outside? Don't feel like cooking? You'll adore this velvety, no-cook avocado soup. It's fresh, nourishing, and quick—and prepared just like a smoothie! Though you may be tempted to dunk tortilla chips into it, think of it as an appetizer soup, and slurp up its creamy goodness with a spoon. You'll love its versatility, too. For special occasions, impress guests' palates with this delightful soup as an amuse-bouche (impromptu meal starter) for 6 or 8 people in mini bowls or espresso cups. (Hint: Serve it slightly warmed, if you prefer.)

SERVES: 3 | SERVING SIZE: ¾ cup
PREP TIME: 12 minutes | COOK TIME: 0 minutes

- 1 large, fully-ripened, Hass avocado, quartered, pitted, and peeled
- 3 tablespoons packed, fresh cilantro leaves with tender stems, divided
- 1 scallion, green part only, chopped
- 1 small garlic clove, chopped
- Juice and ½ lime (1 tablespoon)
- Juice of ½ small lemon (1 tablespoon)
- ½ teaspoon sea salt, or to taste
- ⅛ teaspoon ground coriander

- ⅛ teaspoon ground cumin or cayenne pepper
- 1 ⅓ cups low-sodium vegetable broth, or as needed
- 1 tablespoon pomegranate arils or extra-thinly sliced red-hot chili pepper

DIRECTIONS

1. Add the avocado, 2 tablespoons of the cilantro, the scallion, garlic, lime juice, lemon juice, salt, coriander, cumin, and broth to a blender. Cover and purée on high speed until velvety smooth, at least 2 minutes. Add more broth by the tablespoon if desire a thinner consistency.
2. Transfer the soup to individual small bowls, top with the pomegranate arils and remaining cilantro, and serve.

NUTRITION INFO

Choices/Exchanges: 1 vegetable, 2 fat

Per serving: 110 calories, 8 g total fat, 1 g saturated fat, 0 g trans fat, 0 mg cholesterol, 480 mg sodium, 314 mg potassium, 9 g total carbohydrate, 5 g dietary fiber, 2 g sugars, 0 g added sugars, 2 g protein, 35 mg phosphorus

Avocado Soup Garnishes

This cool and creamy soup is beautifully garnished with fresh cilantro and pomegranate arils or red-hot chili pepper slices. You can also rethink the garnish based on how fancy or not-so-fancy you want to be—or to closely pair it with the meal you're serving. So, top this lovely soup with diced or sliced avocado, lemon or lime zest, roasted pepitas, pistachios, hot pepper sauce, vegan bacon bits, tortilla chips, or whole-grain croutons.

SIMPLE GAZPACHO

Name one thing that makes tomatoes so tasty when they're fully ripened: umami. It's one of the basic tastes (which include sweet, salty, sour, and bitter) that many call "savory." And when tomatoes are fresh, seasonal, and fully ripened, they're ideal for making gazpacho—a perky and pretty soup that's served cool. This raw (no cook!) soup is a taste-bud treat for those who want fine food fast.

SERVES: 4 I SERVING SIZE: 1 cup
PREP TIME: 12 minutes I COOK TIME: 0 minutes

- 5 medium vine-ripened tomatoes, seeded and coarsely chopped
- 1 (5.5-ounce) can spicy vegetable or tomato juice, chilled
- 3 scallions, green and white parts, thinly sliced, divided
- 2 large garlic cloves, minced
- Juice of 1 lime (2 tablespoons)
- 2 teaspoons extra-virgin olive oil
- ¼ teaspoon freshly ground black pepper

DIRECTIONS

1. Purée the tomatoes, vegetable juice, half of the scallions, the garlic, lime juice, and oil in a blender on low speed until just combined. (If your blender has less than a 5-cup capacity, purée in 2 batches.)
2. Pour into small bowls, sprinkle with the pepper and remaining scallions, and serve chilled or at room temperature.

NUTRITION INFO
Choices/Exchanges: 2 vegetable
Per serving: 60 calories, 2.5 g total fat, 0 g saturated fat, 0 g trans fat, 0 mg cholesterol, 85 mg sodium, 462 mg potassium, 9 g total carbohydrate, 2 g dietary fiber, 5 g sugars, 0 g added sugars, 2 g protein, 39 mg phosphorus

Party Twist

This vibrant gazpacho is a party-friendly soup. Double or triple the recipe and purée in batches in Step 1. As a bonus, this gazpacho is tasty served cool or at room temperature, so there's no need to worry about proper timing. Serve this like a punch on a buffet table or at the dining table for more "wow" factor.

See you Later, Tomato Seeds

Pulpy tomato seeds can make a dish a bit bitter or slightly too juicy, which is why you may want to remove them for select recipes, such as this for gazpacho. To remove them, cut the top part off of each tomato crosswise, far enough down to expose its seeded sections. Squeeze the tomatoes by hand to allow the seeds to release and/or use a tiny spoon to scoop them out of each section. That's all there is to it. Think about how you'd like to use the seeds elsewhere, like in a vinaigrette dressing.

RED ONION SOUP WITH SHIITAKE BROTH

I got hooked on French onion soup after I was lucky enough to slurp my first real bowl of it in France over 25 years ago. I wanted to enjoy it at home in a more healthful way, so I created this hearty, onion-loaded, mushroom broth-based version that doesn't need to be laden with cheese. The umami ("meaty" taste) from the shiitakes creates such a savory broth. If you're like me, you'll find this recipe to be more enjoyable than the extra-cheesy, beef broth-based original.

SERVES: 5 I SERVING SIZE: 1 cup
PREP TIME: 16 minutes I COOK TIME: 43 minutes

- 1 tablespoon avocado oil or sunflower oil
- 3 large red onions, halved and thinly sliced
- 2 teaspoons white balsamic or apple cider vinegar
- ½ teaspoon + ⅛ teaspoon sea salt, or to taste
- 1 cup fresh thinly sliced shiitake mushrooms, stems removed
- 1 (32-fluid ounce) carton low-sodium vegetable broth
- ½ teaspoon freshly ground black pepper, or to taste
- 1½ teaspoons minced fresh rosemary
- 1 teaspoon finely chopped fresh thyme leaves + 5 fresh thyme sprigs
- 10 whole-grain pita chips or small, seed-based crackers
- ⅓ cup shredded, plant-based Swiss-style or other plant-based cheese* (1 ounce)

**Note: Ideally, choose vegan cheese products based on tree nuts.*

DIRECTIONS

1. Heat the oil in a stick-resistant stockpot or extra-large saucepan over medium heat. Add the onions, vinegar, and ⅛ teaspoon of the salt and cook while stirring occasionally until softened, about 10 minutes. Increase heat to medium-high, add the mushrooms, and sauté until the onions are well-caramelized, about 15 minutes. Add the broth, the remaining ½ teaspoon salt, the pepper, rosemary, and the chopped thyme, and bring

to a boil over high heat. Reduce heat to low, cover, and simmer until the flavors are developed, about 10 minutes. Meanwhile, preheat the oven to 500°.

2. Place 5 ovenproof soup bowls or crocks onto a baking sheet. Adjust seasoning and ladle the soup into each bowl. Place two of the pita chips on top of each and sprinkle with the plant-based cheese. Bake in the oven on the top oven rack until the cheese is bubbly, about 4 minutes.
3. Garnish each with a thyme sprig, and serve.

NUTRITION INFO

Choices/Exchanges: ½ starch, 2 vegetable, 1 fat

Per serving: 130 calories, 6 g total fat, 2g saturated fat, 0 g trans fat, 0 mg cholesterol, 500 mg sodium, 183 mg potassium, 19 g total carbohydrate, 3 g dietary fiber, 6 g sugars, 0 g added sugars, 3 g protein, 44 mg phosphorus

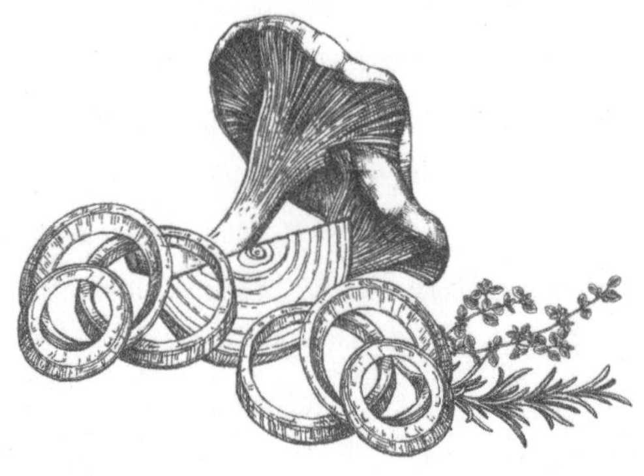

ROASTED ORANGE BELL PEPPER SOUP

I find creamy soups to be like a big warm hug. How about you? The only problem is that a creamy texture typically means a soup is a bit too heavy on the heavy cream and its artery-clogging saturated fat. But this soup provides all of the creaminess that your taste buds dream about in a much better-for-you way. White beans are puréed into the soup to create its distinctive velvetiness. Not only does this soup satisfy your palate, it's a treat for your eyes. The vivid deep-orange color is stunning.

SERVES: 6 | SERVING SIZE: 1 cup
PREP TIME: 15 minutes | COOK TIME: 55 minutes

- 3 large orange or red bell peppers, cut into 4 or 5 pieces each, stems and seeds removed
- 1½ tablespoons extra-virgin olive oil
- 1 large Vidalia or other sweet onion, sliced
- 1½ teaspoons white balsamic or champagne vinegar
- 1 large garlic clove, chopped
- 1 (32–fluid-ounce) carton low-sodium vegetable broth
- 1 (15-ounce) can no-salt-added cannellini or other white beans, drained
- 1¼ teaspoons sea salt
- ½ teaspoon freshly ground black pepper
- 1½ teaspoons fresh thyme or oregano leaves, divided

DIRECTIONS

1. Preheat the broiler. Arrange the bell pepper pieces in a single layer, skin side up, on a baking sheet. Broil until the pepper skins are well charred, about 8 minutes. Transfer bell pepper pieces to a bowl, cover, and let stand until cool enough to handle. Rub off the charred skin.
2. Heat the oil in a Dutch oven or large saucepan over medium heat. Add the onion and vinegar, cover, and cook, stirring twice, until the onion is softened, about 8 minutes. Increase heat to medium high and sauté the onions uncovered until caramelized, about 8 minutes. Add the garlic and sauté until fragrant, about 1 minute. Stir in the bell pepper pieces, broth, beans, salt, black pepper, and 1 teaspoon of the thyme and bring to

a boil. Cover, reduce heat to medium low, and simmer until the bell peppers are very tender, stirring twice, about 25 minutes.

3. Carefully purée the soup in batches in a blender (using the "hot fill" or "liquid" line as a guide) until smooth. Alternatively, blend in the saucepan using an immersion blender.
4. Ladle the soup into bowls, sprinkle with the remaining ½ teaspoon thyme, and serve.

NUTRITION INFO
Choices/Exchanges: 1 starch, 2 vegetable, 1 fat
Per serving: 190 calories, 4.5 g total fat, 0.5 g saturated fat, 0 g trans fat, 0 mg cholesterol, 590 mg sodium, 575 mg potassium, 30 g total carbohydrate, 10 g dietary fiber, 7 g sugars, 0 g added sugars, 8 g protein, 155 mg phosphorus

Why Eat Beans?

One of the many reasons is that they provide soluble fiber, which can help keep you feeling full between meals. Basically, after you eat a meal rich in soluble fiber, signals are sent from your gut to your brain, resulting in the release of sugar from foods over longer periods of time instead of all at once. So boost your bean intake. Beans can be eaten in salads, salsa, sides, and more. They're beneficial including when puréed into a soup, like in this recipe, too.

BROCCOLI FLORETS AND STEMS CASHEW CRÈME SOUP

If you're a fan of creamy, cheesy broccoli soup, this recipe is for you! It's got all of the creaminess that you'll desire thanks to the cashews that become velvety when blended. You'll get that intriguing touch of "cheesiness" from the nutritional yeast flakes. And you'll enjoy all of the broccoli goodness from, of course, broccoli! This golden-hued soup is not just a bowl of nutritiousness, it's loaded with deliciousness.

SERVES: 6 | SERVING SIZE: 1 cup
PREP TIME: 18 minutes | COOK TIME: 40 minutes

- 1 tablespoon extra-virgin olive or avocado oil
- 16 ounces fresh broccoli florets and sliced non-woody stems (about 5 cups packed)
- 1 medium yellow onion, chopped
- 1 large garlic clove, minced
- 1 (32-ounce) carton low-sodium vegetable broth
- ½ cup unsalted, unroasted cashews
- ¾ teaspoon sea salt, or to taste
- ¼ teaspoon freshly ground pepper
- ⅛ teaspoon ground nutmeg
- 1 tablespoon nutritional yeast flakes
- Juice of ½ small lemon (1 tablespoon), or to taste

DIRECTIONS

1. Heat the oil in a stockpot or extra-large saucepan over medium-high heat. Add the broccoli florets and stems and onion and cook while stirring occasionally until the florets are bright green and onion is caramelized (browned), about 8 minutes. Add the garlic and sauté until fragrant, about 30 seconds.
2. Add the broth, cashews, salt, pepper, and nutmeg and bring to a boil over high heat. Cover, reduce heat to low, and simmer until the broccoli stems are fork tender, about 30 minutes. Stir in the nutritional yeast and lemon juice.
3. In batches, purée the soup in a blender on high speed using the "hot fill" or "liquid" line as a guide until velvety smooth, about 1 minute per batch. Return the puréed soup to a clean pot over low heat. Adjust seasoning.
4. Ladle into bowls and serve.

NUTRITION INFO

Choices/Exchanges: 2 vegetable, 2 fat

Per serving: 140 calories, 8 g total fat, 1.5 g saturated fat, 0 g trans fat, 0 mg cholesterol, 410 mg sodium, 373 mg potassium, 13 g total carbohydrate, 4 g dietary fiber, 4 g sugars, 0 g added sugars, 6 g protein, 124 mg phosphorus

Broccoli Soup Toppers

No garnish is required for this comforting bowl of yum. But if you want to add a bit more eye appeal or go a little glam, try these ideas at serving time. Swirl in plant-based sour cream; top with vegan bacon bits, plant-based Cheddar-style cheese, or sautéed small broccoli florets; or sprinkle with grated nutmeg and hot pepper flakes.

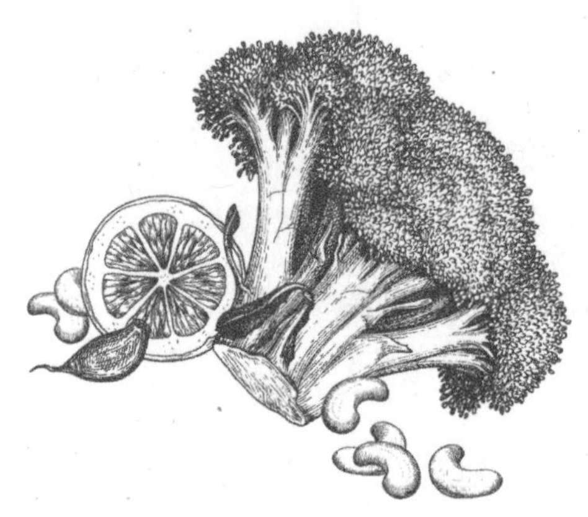

BLACK BEAN, POBLANO, AND TORTILLA SOUP

If you're a Mexican cuisine aficionada or aficionado, you'll want this highly flavored, tomato-based soup at the top of your list. The crushed roasted tomatoes provide lots of umami (savoriness), plus a punch of health-protective lycopene, which is a carotenoid that may help to reduce oxidative stress in people with type 2 diabetes. The black beans make it exceptionally satisfying and extra nutritious. And the topping of crisp tortilla chips, creamy avocado, and zingy lime zest make it joyful.

SERVES: 6 I SERVING SIZE: 1 cup
PREP TIME: 22 minutes I COOK TIME: 28 minutes

- 2 teaspoons unrefined peanut or avocado oil
- 1 medium poblano pepper, finely diced
- 1 small or ½ large white onion, finely diced
- Juice and zest of 1 lime (2 tablespoons juice), divided
- ½ teaspoon sea salt, divided
- 1 small jalapeño pepper, with some seeds, minced
- 2 large garlic cloves, minced
- 1 (32-fluid-ounce) carton low-sodium vegetable broth
- 1 (15-ounce) can no-salt-added black beans, drained
- 1 (14.5-ounce) can crushed roasted tomatoes (1¾ cups)
- 1 teaspoon finely chopped fresh oregano leaves
- ¼ teaspoon ground cumin, or to taste
- ¼ cup chopped fresh cilantro
- 12 unsalted yellow or white corn tortilla chips, coarsely broken
- 1 Hass avocado, pitted, peeled, diced

DIRECTIONS

1. Heat the oil in a stockpot or Dutch oven over medium-high heat. Add the poblano pepper, onion, 2 teaspoons of the lime juice, and ¼ teaspoon of the salt and sauté until the onion is lightly caramelized, about 8 minutes. Add the jalapeño and garlic and sauté for 1 minute. Add the broth, beans, tomatoes, oregano, cumin, and the remaining ¼

teaspoon salt and bring to a boil over high heat. Reduce heat to medium and simmer, uncovered, until the poblano peppers are fully softened, about 15 minutes.

2. Remove from heat. Stir in the cilantro and the remaining lime juice. Adjust seasoning.
3. Ladle into bowls, top with tortilla chips, avocado, and desired amount of the lime zest, and serve.

NUTRITION INFO

Choices/Exchanges: 1 starch, 1½ vegetable, 1 fat

Per serving: 170 calories, 6 g total fat, 1 g saturated fat, 0 g trans fat, 0 mg cholesterol, 390 mg sodium, 540 mg potassium, 25 g total carbohydrate, 8 g dietary fiber, 5 g sugars, 0 g added sugars, 6 g protein, 110 mg phosphorus

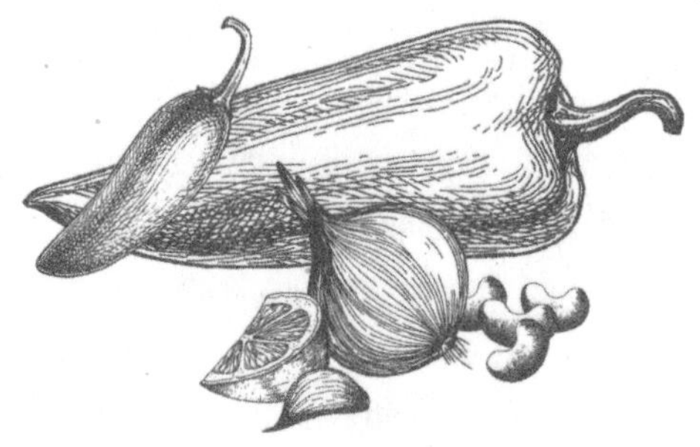

GARLIC SPINACH DAL STEW

Dal refers to split pulses, like lentils. It also refers to a soup or other dish made with them, like this tangy lentil-based stew. Its rich South Asian goodness—with a spice trio of cumin, coriander, and turmeric—will awaken your taste buds. And the pops of color and flavor from the grape tomatoes and fresh baby spinach create extra appeal. Though you can slurp on this stew any time of year, you'll definitely want to savor it around the winter holidays when those pops of red and green provide festive delight.

SERVES: 6 | SERVING SIZE: 1 cup
PREP TIME: 20 minutes | COOK TIME: 45 minutes

- 2 teaspoons extra-virgin olive oil
- 1 medium red onion, diced
- 2 large stalks celery, diced
- 1 small serrano pepper, with seeds, minced
- Juice and zest of 1 lemon (3 tablespoons juice)
- ¾ teaspoons sea salt, divided
- 3 large garlic cloves, thinly sliced or minced
- 5 cups low-sodium vegetable broth
- ¾ cup dried, French green lentils, rinsed and drained
- 1 pint grape tomatoes
- ½ teaspoon + ⅛ teaspoon *South Asian Spice Trio* (following)
- ½ teaspoon freshly ground black pepper, or to taste
- 5 cups packed fresh baby spinach (5 ounces)
- ¼ cup plain unsweetened plant-based Greek-style yogurt (optional)

DIRECTIONS

1. Heat the oil in a stockpot over medium-high heat. Add the onion, celery, serrano pepper, lemon juice, and ¼ teaspoon of the salt and sauté until the onion is softened and lightly caramelized, about 8 minutes. Add the garlic and sauté for 30 seconds.
2. Add the broth, lentils, tomatoes, spice mixture, black pepper, and the remaining ½ teaspoon salt and bring to a boil over high heat. Reduce heat to medium-low and simmer, uncovered, until the lentils are tender, about 30 minutes. Stir in the spinach and simmer until the spinach is wilted, about 2 minutes. And, if using, stir in the plant-based yogurt.
3. Ladle into individual bowls, sprinkle with desired amount of the lemon zest, and serve.

NUTRITION INFO
Choices/Exchanges: 1 starch, 1 vegetable, ½ fat
Per serving: 130 calories, 2.5 g total fat, 0 g saturated fat, 0 g trans fat, 0 mg cholesterol, 450 mg sodium, 540 mg potassium, 22 g total carbohydrate, 6 g dietary fiber, 5 g sugars, 0 g added sugars, 7 g protein, 40 mg phosphorus

SOUTH ASIAN SPICE TRIO

Makes 5 servings, 1 teaspoon each

- 2 teaspoons ground cumin*
- 2 teaspoons ground coriander*
- 1 teaspoon ground turmeric

Stir together the cumin, coriander, and turmeric. Store in a labeled jar. Makes 5 teaspoons. Use in *Garlic Spinach Dal Stew* and other recipes of choice.

**Hint: Instead of buying ground spices, toast whole cumin and coriander seeds and then grind in a coffee grinder or peppermill for a warmer, earthier flavor.*

NUTRITION INFO
Choices/Exchanges: 0
Per serving: 15 calories, 0 g total fat, 0 g saturated fat, 0 g trans fat, 0 mg cholesterol, 0 mg sodium, 20 mg potassium, 1 g total carbohydrate, 0 g dietary fiber, 0 g sugars, 0 g added sugars, 0 g protein, 5 mg phosphorus

TUSCAN VEGETABLE STEW

Here's a hearty vegetable stew that will be enjoyed by all, especially veggie lovers. And if you're not already a vegetable lover, it might just turn you into one. This is a tasty bowlful of contrasting textures and colors and so much wholesomeness. It's inspired by the iconic Tuscan stew *Ribollita* but simpler, carb-friendlier, and herbier.

SERVES: 6 I SERVING SIZE: 1 cup
PREP TIME: 20 minutes I COOK TIME: 40 minutes

- 1 tablespoon extra-virgin olive oil
- 1 small or ½ large red onion, chopped
- 1¼ teaspoons sea salt, divided
- 2 large garlic cloves, minced
- 1 (15-ounce) can no-salt-added cannellini or other white beans, drained, divided
- 3½ cups low-sodium vegetable broth, divided
- 6 cups chopped organic lacinato kale or savoy cabbage (6 ounces)
- 1 pint grape tomatoes
- 2 teaspoons finely chopped fresh rosemary
- ¾ teaspoon freshly ground black pepper
- 2½ ounces day-old, whole-grain bread, cut into ¾-inch cubes
- ½ cup chopped, fresh, flat-leaf parsley

DIRECTIONS

1. Heat the oil in a stockpot over medium heat. Add the onion and ¼ teaspoon of the salt and cook, stirring occasionally, until the onion is softened, about 8 minutes. Add the garlic and sauté until fragrant, about 1 minute.
2. Meanwhile, add half of the beans and ¾ cup of the broth to a blender or food processor. Cover and blend until smooth.
3. Add the bean purée, kale, tomatoes, rosemary, pepper, and the remaining 2¾ cups broth and 1 teaspoon salt to the stockpot and bring to a boil over high heat. Reduce heat to medium low and simmer, covered, until the kale is tender, about 20 minutes. Stir in the bread, parsley, and the remaining beans, and simmer, uncovered, for 5 minutes to complete the cooking process.
4. Ladle into individual bowls and serve.

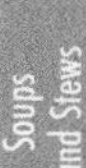

NUTRITION INFO

Choices/Exchanges 1½ starch, 1 vegetable, 1 lean protein

Per serving: 200 calories, 4.5 g total fat, 1 g saturated fat, 0 g trans fat, 0 mg cholesterol, 590 mg sodium, 855 mg potassium, 31 g total carbohydrate, 7 g dietary fiber, 3 g sugars, 0 g added sugars, 13 g protein, 195 mg phosphorus

At the Table

If you enjoy high-flavored extras or want to make this more luxurious for a special occasion, try one or more of these ideas when serving this stew. Drizzle individual servings with a little extra-virgin olive oil for bonus richness. Sprinkle with freshly grated plant-based Parmesan-style cheese for an extra pop of savoriness. Squirt with lemon wedges for citrusy fragrance and zing. Or, for a casual family-friendly gathering, plop in prepared plant-based Italian meatballs or sausage slices.

INDIAN SWEET POTATO EDAMAME STEW

You'll be enamored with this entrée-sized stew, especially if you're a fan of Indian flavors. Not yet an Indian cuisine enthusiast? This satiating stew is a scrumptious starting point. The cinnamon and coriander provide a just-right worldly accent to the large bites of sweet potatoes and the unique addition of protein-packed edamame. The cilantro goes beyond a regular garnish and adds freshness at serving time.

SERVES: 5 | SERVING SIZE: 1 ⅔ cups
PREP TIME: 18 minutes | COOK TIME: 1 hour 8 minutes

- 2 teaspoon extra-virgin olive oil
- 1 large white onion, cut into large dices
- 2 large garlic cloves, minced
- 1 teaspoon harissa or ¼ teaspoon hot pepper sauce, or to taste
- ¾ teaspoon ground cinnamon
- ¾ teaspoon ground coriander
- 1 (15-ounce) can diced tomatoes (with liquid)
- 3 medium-large (9-ounce) sweet potatoes, unpeeled, root ends trimmed, cut into 1-inch cubes (8 cups cubes)
- 2 cups low-sodium vegetable broth
- ½ teaspoon freshly ground black pepper, or to taste
- 1½ cups thawed, frozen, shelled organic edamame
- ½ teaspoon sea salt, or to taste
- ¼ cup roughly chopped fresh cilantro, or to taste

DIRECTIONS

1. Heat the oil in a stockpot or Dutch oven over medium-high heat. Add the onion and sauté until lightly caramelized, about 8 minutes. Add the garlic, harissa, cinnamon, and coriander and sauté for 30 seconds. Add the tomatoes with liquid, sweet potatoes, broth, and black pepper and bring to a boil over high heat. Reduce heat to low, cover, and simmer until the sweet potatoes are cooked through and softened, about 45 minutes.

2. Stir in the edamame and salt and continue to simmer, covered, until the edamame is fully heated, about 10 minutes. Adjust seasoning.
3. Ladle the stew into a bowl, sprinkle with the cilantro, and serve.

NUTRITION INFO

Choices/Exchanges: 2 starch, 1½ vegetable, 1 lean protein

Per serving: 250 calories, 4.5 g total fat, 0.5 g saturated fat, 0 g trans fat, 0 mg cholesterol, 570 mg sodium, 770 mg potassium, 44 g total carbohydrate, 9 g dietary fiber, 12 g sugars, 0 g added sugars, 9 g protein, 160 mg phosphorus

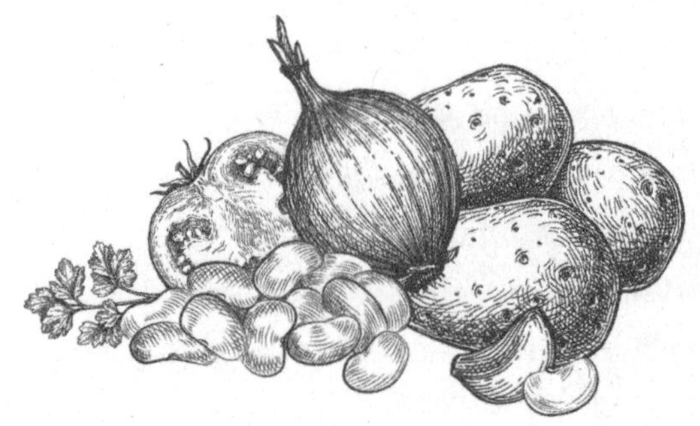

CALIFORNIA CANNELLINI CHILI

Not your ordinary chili! You'll use white beans, cinnamon, and a topping of avocado, which makes this version special for all tastes. A little splash of freshly squeezed orange juice with its fibrous pulp provides a perfect accent of natural sweetness. Want to make this chili still more special? As an ode to San Francisco, enjoy individual servings in hollowed-out, whole-grain sourdough bread rolls, if you have room for the carbs.

SERVES: 8 | SERVING SIZE: 1 cup
PREP TIME: 20 minutes | COOK TIME: 28 minutes

- 1 tablespoon avocado oil or unrefined peanut oil
- 1 large red onion, finely diced
- 1 large green bell pepper, finely diced
- 1 tablespoon white balsamic or white wine vinegar
- ¾ teaspoon sea salt, divided
- 2 large garlic cloves, minced
- 1 (14.5-ounce) can crushed roasted tomatoes (1¾ cups)
- 3 cups low-sodium vegetable broth
- ⅓ cup freshly squeezed orange juice with pulp or pear nectar
- 1 tablespoon + 1 teaspoon chili powder, or to taste
- ½ teaspoon ground cinnamon, or to taste
- ½ teaspoon freshly ground black pepper, or to taste
- 2 (15-ounce) cans no-salt-added cannellini or other white beans, drained (3 cups)
- ⅓ cup shredded plant-based Monterey Jack-style cheese or vegan cheese crumbles*
- 1 small Hass avocado, peeled, pitted, and finely diced
- 2 tablespoons roughly chopped fresh cilantro

**Note: Ideally, choose vegan cheese products based on tree nuts.*

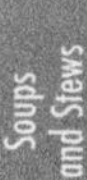

DIRECTIONS

1. Heat the oil in a stockpot over medium-high heat. Add the onion, bell pepper, vinegar, and ¼ teaspoon of the salt and sauté until the onion is lightly caramelized, about 8 minutes. Add the garlic and sauté for 1 minute.

2. Stir in the tomatoes, broth, orange juice with pulp, chili powder, cinnamon, black pepper, and the remaining ½ teaspoon salt and bring to a boil over high heat. Reduce heat to medium-low, stir in the beans, and simmer, uncovered, until desired consistency, about 15 minutes. Adjust seasoning.
3. Ladle the chili into individual bowls. Sprinkle with the plant-based cheese, avocado, and cilantro, and serve.

NUTRITION INFO

Choices/Exchanges: 1 starch, 2 vegetable, 1 fat

Per serving: 180 calories, 6 g total fat, 1.5 g saturated fat, 0 g trans fat, 0 mg cholesterol, 450 mg sodium, 704 mg potassium, 26 g total carbohydrate, 8 g dietary fiber, 6 g sugars, 0 g added sugars, 7 g protein, 97 mg phosphorus

Water Method to Keep a Cut Avocado Fresh

Only need part of an avocado for a recipe? Once cut open, it will begin to brown. To help prevent discoloration, place the unused portion cut side down in a sealable glass container or jar, fully cover with cold water, seal and store in the fridge for up to 3 days. If it does discolor, all you need to do is slice off the top layer. (Hint: When possible, keep the seed in the avocado to help better protect the portion where the seed sits.)

SPICY GAME-DAY CHILI

Yes, you can have game-day grub. This nicely spiced chili can be a highlight of any gathering. The cocoa powder and pumpkin pie spice create flavor intrigue. The cauliflower provides extra body in a healthy way. If you can find purple cauliflower, pick it up. It contains anthocyanins, which have shown promise in reducing risk of type 2 diabetes, heart disease, cancer, and more. Simmer the chili until it's soupy or extra-thick—it's up to you. Either way, this cup of comfort is perfect as is, though awesome when topped with guac too!

SERVES: 8 | SERVING SIZE: 1 cup
PREP TIME: 20 minutes | COOK TIME: 28 to 31 minutes

- 1 tablespoon sunflower or avocado oil
- 3 cups finely chopped purple or white cauliflower florets
- 1 large yellow onion, finely diced
- 2 teaspoons apple cider vinegar
- ¾ teaspoon sea salt, divided
- 1 small jalapeño pepper, with some seeds, minced
- 2 large garlic cloves, minced
- 1 (32-fluid ounce) carton low-sodium vegetable broth
- 1 (14.5-ounce) can crushed, roasted tomatoes (1¾ cups)
- 1½ tablespoons chili powder, or to taste
- 2 teaspoons unsweetened cocoa powder
- ½ teaspoon ground pumpkin pie spice or cinnamon, or to taste
- 1 (15-ounce) can no-salt-added red kidney or black beans, drained (1½ cups)
- ¼ cup plant-based sour cream
- 2 tablespoons roughly chopped fresh flat-leaf parsley or minced fresh chives

DIRECTIONS

1. Heat the oil in a stockpot over medium-high heat. Add the cauliflower, onion, vinegar, and ¼ teaspoon of the salt and sauté until the onion begins to caramelize, about 8 minutes. Add the jalapeño and garlic and sauté until fragrant, about 30 seconds.

2. Stir in the broth, tomatoes, chili powder, cocoa powder, pumpkin pie spice, and the remaining ½ teaspoon salt and bring to a boil over high heat. Reduce heat to medium-low, stir in the beans and simmer, uncovered, until desired consistency, about 15 to 18 minutes. Adjust seasoning.
3. Ladle the chili into individual bowls, top with the plant-based sour cream, sprinkle with the parsley, and serve.

NUTRITION INFO

Choices/Exchanges: ½ starch, 2 vegetable

Per serving: 100 calories, 3.5 g total fat, 0.5 g saturated fat, 0 g trans fat, 0 mg cholesterol, 440 mg sodium, 511 mg potassium, 19 g total carbohydrate, 7 g dietary fiber, 5 g sugars, 0 g added sugars, 6 g protein, 96 mg phosphorus

Game-Day Gathering Serving Tip

One fun way to serve this chili on football game day is along with a buffet of colorful toppings, like diced green bell pepper, diced red onion, diced tomato, lime wedges, pumpkin seeds, tortilla strips, plant-based sour cream, and guacamole. For an extra dose of entertainment, enjoy the chili ladled over pulse-based or whole-grain spaghetti, which is considered Cincinnati-style chili ("two-way"). Make it a "three-way" by sprinkling it with plant-based cheese, or a "four-way" by adding diced onions.

Desserts and Drinks

JUST PEACHY BOWLS

These gorgeous "bowls" look impressive, but they're so simple to make. The topping is plant-based, Greek-style yogurt that you'll sweeten naturally with mashed banana. You won't need a whole banana, so slice the rest and freeze for later. The plant-based, Greek-style yogurt provides a luxuriously creamy mouthfeel. Before adding banana, you can strain it in a cheesecloth- or unbleached paper towel-lined mesh strainer to make it a little thicker. Or you can slightly freeze it, stir it, and scoop it up like soft serve. Either way, when dolloped over juicy peaches, the result is divine—especially when the fruit is at its peak in the spring or summer.

SERVES: 4 | SERVING SIZE: 1 bowl (½ peach with topping)
PREP TIME: 8 minutes | COOK TIME: 0 minutes (if using pre-toasted or roasted nuts)

- 3 tablespoons fully mashed ripe banana (or banana baby food!)
- 1 cup vanilla, unsweetened, plant-based, Greek-style yogurt
- 2 large fully ripened peaches, halved, pits and stems removed
- 2 tablespoons natural sliced almonds, pan-toasted, or roasted pistachios
- 20 small fresh mint leaves

DIRECTIONS

1. In a mixer bowl, blend the banana with an electric mixer until fully whipped, then mix in the yogurt until velvety smooth. Alternatively stir together the plant-based yogurt and banana in a small bowl until creamy smooth.
2. Place each peach half onto a small plate, cut-side up. Top each half with the plant-based yogurt mixture, almonds, and mint, and serve.

NUTRITION INFO

Choices/Exchanges: 1 fruit, 1 lean protein

Per serving: 110 calories, 4 g total fat, 0 g saturated fat, 0 g trans fat, 0 mg cholesterol, 60 mg sodium, 306 mg potassium, 13 g total carbohydrate, 2 g dietary fiber, 8 g sugars, 0 g added sugars, 8 g protein, 34 mg phosphorus

Flavorful Variations

Lightly brush the peach halves with avocado oil or sunflower oil, or spritz them with organic oil cooking spray, and grill until grill markings form. It'll make this dessert uniquely sweet and smoky. Also, mix and match these refreshing bowls. Try various fresh seasonal fruit halves and add different flavorings to the plant-based, Greek-style yogurt mixture, such as pure almond extract, citrus zest, or fresh mashed berries of choice.

DARK CHOCOLATE RASPBERRY PUDDING

There's no dairy in this luscious chocolate pudding. Whipped avocado creates the thick, rich, and super creamy texture. The sweetness comes naturally from fruit jam—with or without seeds. The classic combination of raspberry and chocolate is a delight. (Hint: If you're passionate about dark chocolate, add another tablespoon of unsweetened cocoa powder to the recipe.) And the use of sea salt makes this a true taste winner. Ideally make this the day before you want to enjoy it to allow flavors to marry. A mouthwatering vegan dessert creation!

SERVES: 2 | SERVING SIZE: about ½ cup
PREP TIME: 10 minutes (plus chilling time) | COOK TIME: 0 minutes

- 1 large fully ripened Hass avocado, peeled and pitted
- 3 tablespoons fruit-sweetened raspberry or black raspberry fruit spread (jam), or to taste*
- 2 tablespoons unsweetened cocoa powder
- ½ teaspoon pure vanilla extract
- ¼ teaspoon + ⅛ teaspoon sea salt
- ¼ teaspoon raspberry-flavored red wine vinegar or aged balsamic vinegar
- 6 fresh or thawed frozen raspberries

**Note: Ideally, choose a fruit spread without added sugars.*

DIRECTIONS

1. Place the avocado, jam, cocoa powder, vanilla extract, salt, and vinegar in a food processor or the bowl of an electric mixer. Blend until smooth and fluffy, about 2 minutes, scraping down the sides as needed. Adjust ingredients, if needed.
2. Transfer the pudding to small dessert dishes. Chill for at least 1 hour (or, ideally, overnight) to allow flavors to mingle. Top with the raspberries and serve.

NUTRITION INFO
Choices/Exchanges: 1 carbohydrate, 2 fat
Per serving: 170 calories, 11 g total fat, 2 g saturated fat, 0 g trans fat, 0 mg cholesterol, 450 mg sodium, 435 mg potassium, 20 g total carbohydrate, 8 g dietary fiber, 9 g sugars, 0 g added sugars, 2 g protein, 80 mg phosphorus

Avocado Facts

Better sex is why the Aztecs supposedly loved the avocado—the "forbidden fruit." It's also called the "alligator pear." But most folks love its luscious texture, taste, and versatility regardless of its name or reputation. The Hass avocado is the most popular of California's seven top varieties, including Fuerte, Bacon, Reed, Lamb Hass, Zutano, and Pinkerton..

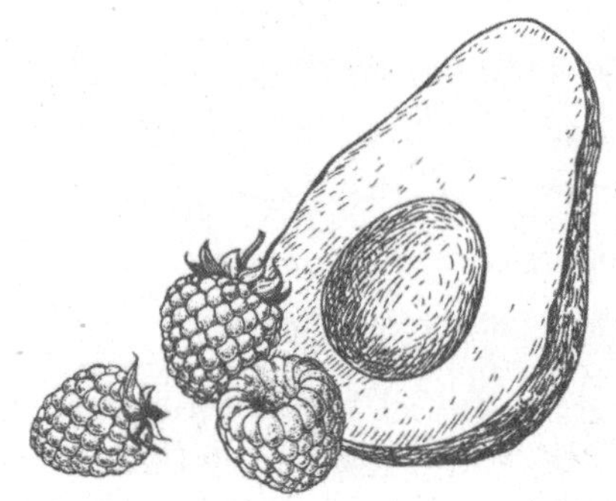

WHIPPED BANANA SHERBET

A banana doesn't seem much like a dessert. But when that banana is frozen and whirled with fresh lemon juice, pure flavor extracts, and unsweetened plant-based milk, it transforms into a sweet, frozen treat. This sherbet assures that you'll be making your sugar calories count. When sugar comes naturally in the form of fruit, you're getting deliciousness along with quality nutrition, including dietary fiber. So, gather these ingredients and whip . . . whip it good!

SERVES: 4 I SERVING SIZE: ½ cup
PREP TIME: 6 minutes (plus freezing time) I COOK TIME: 0 minutes

- 3 medium fully ripened bananas, peeled, sliced, and frozen
- 1 teaspoon fresh lemon juice
- 1 teaspoon pure vanilla extract
- ⅛ teaspoon pure almond extract
- ½ cup plain, unsweetened coconut milk beverage or plant-based milk of choice

DIRECTIONS

1. Purée the frozen banana slices, lemon juice, extracts, and coconut milk beverage in a blender or food processor until very smooth. Add additional milk beverage by tablespoonfuls only if necessary.
2. Pour the banana purée into 4 small, chilled glass dessert bowls. Serve immediately, soft-serve style. Or cover and freeze for 2 hours, or until solid, and serve.

NUTRITION INFO
Choices/Exchanges: 1½ fruit
Per serving: 90 calories, 1 g total fat, 0.5 g saturated fat, 0 g trans fat, 0 mg cholesterol, 0 mg sodium, 330 mg potassium, 21 g total carbohydrate, 2 g dietary fiber, 11 g sugars, 0 g added sugars, 1 g protein, 20 mg phosphorus

Fresh Fact

When the banana peels are full of tiny brown "freckles," it means the bananas are fully ripened. That's when they're best for use in recipes, like this sherbet. However, if you plan to just eat a banana as is, enjoy it before it freckles, and preferably when it's at least slightly green. When underripe, bananas contain more fiber and resistant starch than when they're fully ripe. Resistant starch passes through your intestines intact, so it may be beneficial for people with or at risk for diabetes since these carbs don't directly break down into sugar. This may curb spikes in blood glucose.

CHOCOLATE PEPPERMINT "NICE CREAM"

What's your favorite flavor duo? Mine is definitely chocolate and mint! So this creamy dessert is dreamy to me. There's no dairy in it, so technically it's not ice cream. The name "nice cream" works like a charm. The main ingredient is banana, which provides its delectable creaminess and sweetness. As you're puréeing the "nice cream," it starts out looking crumbly. But be patient, it'll soon become velvety smooth. Oh, and then there's fun crunch from the cacao nibs—which also provide antioxidants with no added sugars in sight.

SERVES: 3 | SERVING SIZE: about ½ cup
PREP TIME: 10 minutes (plus freezing time) | COOK TIME: 0 minutes

- 2 medium fully ripened bananas, peeled, sliced into coins, and frozen
- 3 tablespoons unsweetened cocoa powder
- ½ teaspoon pure vanilla extract
- ¼ teaspoon pure peppermint extract
- 1 tablespoon cacao nibs

DIRECTIONS

1. Add the frozen banana coins, cocoa powder, and extracts to a food processor. Cover and pulse 10 times to chop the bananas. Then process on high speed until creamy, about 2½ minutes, while stopping and scraping down the inside of the food processor container about every 30 seconds of processing. Add the cacao nibs and pulse 3 times to combine.
2. Enjoy the nice cream immediately, soft-serve style. Or freeze until solid—then at serving time, set it out for 15 minutes to soften, scoop, and serve.

NUTRITION INFO
Choices/Exchanges: 1½ fruit, ½ fat
Per serving: 110 calories, 2.5 g total fat, 1.5 g saturated fat, 0 g trans fat, 0 mg cholesterol, 0 mg sodium, 410 mg potassium, 24 g total carbohydrate, 5 dietary fiber, 11 g sugars, 0 g added sugars, 2 g protein, 70 mg phosphorus

How to Freeze Bananas

Peel the fully ripened bananas. Slice crosswise into coins. Arrange the banana coins on an unbleached parchment paper-lined rimmed baking sheet, cover, and freeze for at least 4 hours or overnight. Use in the recipe. Or transfer the frozen banana coins into a sealable silicone freezer pouch or other container for later use.

What Are Cacao Nibs?

Cacao nibs come from dried cacao beans that grow in football-shaped pods on cacao trees. Yes, chocolate (or at least its key ingredient) comes from a tree! They're called nibs since they're simply cracked up bits of the dried cacao beans, kind of like extra-coarsely ground black pepper. They are on the bitter side since there's no sugar added to them. But they provide all of the best nutrition (hello polyphenols!) of the cacao bean. And they offer a distinct crunchiness in dessert recipes, like cookies or this "nice cream."

OATMEAL COOKIES WITH SEA SALT

Whip up a batch of these new-fashioned favorites and you'll quickly find out that it's possible to have great-tasting cookies with good-for-you ingredients. The oats and whole-wheat pastry flour offer a notable amount of fiber. The coconut sugar has a lower glycemic index than white sugar. Unsweetened applesauce provides bonus sweetness, naturally. And chia seeds act like eggs here. Basically, these cookies will satisfy anyone's "sweet tooth" in a surprisingly nourishing way.

SERVES: 15 | SERVING SIZE: 1 cookie
PREP TIME: 16 minutes | COOK TIME: 18 minutes

- 1 cup old-fashioned oats
- ½ cup whole-wheat pastry flour
- 1¼ teaspoons baking powder
- ½ teaspoon + ⅛ teaspoon sea salt
- Pinch of cinnamon
- 1 cup coconut sugar
- 3 tablespoons vegan butter, room temperature
- ⅓ cup unsweetened applesauce
- 1 tablespoon chia seeds
- 1½ teaspoons pure vanilla extract

DIRECTIONS

1. Preheat the oven to 350°F. Line two baking sheets with silicone baking mats or unbleached parchment paper.
2. In a small bowl, combine the oats, flour, baking powder, salt, and cinnamon.
3. Using an electric mixer at medium speed, blend together the sugar and vegan butter in a mixer bowl into a moist crumbly mixture, at least 1 minute. Add the applesauce, chia seeds, and vanilla, and blend on medium speed until evenly combined. Add the dry mixture and blend on low speed until just combined.
4. Drop the batter using a medium (2-tablespoon) cookie scoop or by fully rounded measuring tablespoon onto the prepared baking sheets to make 7 or 8 cookies each. Bake until browned, about 20 minutes.

5. Remove from the oven and let cool completely on the baking sheets on racks. The cookies will crisp as they cool. Store them in an airtight container at room temperature for up to 3 days—or freeze them for up to 2 months.

NUTRITION INFO

Choices/Exchanges: 1 starch, ½ fat

Per serving: 100 calories, 2.5 g total fat, 2 g saturated fat, 0 g trans fat, 0 mg cholesterol, 130 mg sodium, 86 mg potassium, 18 g total carbohydrate, 3 g dietary fiber, 11 g sugars, 10 g added sugars, 1 g protein, 28 mg phosphorus

Vegan Butter: Did You Know?

Use plant-based butter as a dairy-free alternative to butter, not necessarily as a healthier option. It has a similar mouthfeel and flavor profile. You can use it as an equal swap for butter in recipes since it's based on plant-derived oils; it melts like butter and is mainly fat. Though, since plant-based milk and/or water is added, there might be a slight texture change when using it in large quantities in baking.

Faster Fix

Make your own oatmeal cookie dry mix. Measure the oats, flour, baking powder, salt, and cinnamon into a clean jar. Label it "oatmeal cookie mix" and date it. Store the mix in the pantry up to a couple of months. Then skip Step 2 when ready to bake these cookies

ALMOND COOKIE BALLS

These simple, little, button-like cookies with their perfect hint of sweetness are grain-free, gluten-free, and the perfect after-dinner bite or mini snack. They're also kind of like biscotti, since they're lovely when dunked into your cup of coffee, tea, or sugar-free hot cocoa. Be sure to use almond flour, not almond meal. Store the baked treats in a sealed container in the fridge for a week or the freezer for up to 3 months (though they'll certainly be eaten up well before that!).

SERVES: 12 | SERVING SIZE: 1 cookie
PREP TIME: 8 minutes | COOK TIME: 16 minutes

- 4 ounces almond flour (1 cup)
- 3 tablespoons coconut sugar
- ½ teaspoon baking powder
- ⅛ teaspoon sea salt
- 2 tablespoons unsweetened peppermint tea or cold water
- ¼ teaspoon pure vanilla extract
- ⅛ teaspoon pure almond extract

DIRECTIONS

1. Preheat the oven to 350°F. Line a baking sheet with a silicone baking mat or unbleached parchment paper.
2. In a medium bowl, whisk together the almond flour, coconut sugar, baking powder, and salt until well-combined and no lumps remain.
3. In a liquid measuring cup, stir together the tea and extracts. Pour into the almond flour mixture and stir with a flexible spatula until a dough forms.
4. Roll the dough by hand into 12 balls and place onto the prepared baking sheet. (If desired, pat to slightly flatten into 1¾-inch-diameter cookies.) Bake until golden brown, about 16 minutes.
5. Remove from the oven and let cool for 5 minutes on the baking sheet on a cooling rack. Then transfer the cookies directly to the rack to completely cool and crisp.

NUTRITION INFO

Choices/Exchanges: ½ carbohydrate, 1 fat

Per serving: 70 calories, 4.5 g total fat, 0 g saturated fat, 0 g trans fat, 0 mg cholesterol, 25 mg sodium, 82 mg potassium, 5 g total carbohydrate, 1 g dietary fiber, 3 g sugars, 3 g added sugars, 2 g protein, 46 mg phosphorus

FUDGY PLANT-BASED BROWNIES

Want an occasional chocolatey treat? I've given traditional brownies a semi-extreme makeover here, so they're healthier yet still taste decadent. Most notably, I use beans and applesauce to pump up the fudginess and fiber. Whole-wheat pastry flour and chia seeds add body and still more fiber. As for taste, coconut sugar creates the just-right amount of sweetness in a natural way, while the combination of baking chocolate and cocoa powder provides the luxurious chocolatiness that you expect from brownies. Yum!

SERVES: 16 | SERVING SIZE: 1 brownie
PREP TIME: 17 minutes | COOK TIME: 26 minutes

- ½ cup canned, drained no-salt-added black beans
- 3 tablespoons ground chia seeds or 2 tablespoons whole chia seeds
- ⅔ cup unsweetened applesauce, divided
- 1¼ teaspoons pure vanilla extract
- 1 cup coconut sugar
- ¼ cup avocado oil or sunflower oil
- ½ teaspoon sea salt
- 2½ ounces unsweetened baking chocolate, chopped
- ⅓ cup unsweetened cocoa powder
- 3 ounces whole-wheat pastry flour (⅔ cup)

DIRECTIONS

1. Preheat the oven to 375°F. Set aside an 8-inch square silicone baking pan, or line the bottom of an 8-inch square baking pan with a silicone baking mat or unbleached parchment paper.
2. Add the beans, chia seeds, ⅓ cup of the applesauce, and the vanilla to a blender or food processor. Cover and purée. Transfer to a small bowl and set aside.
3. In a large saucepan, stir together the sugar, oil, salt, and remaining ⅓ cup applesauce. Place over medium-high heat and cook, while stirring, until the mixture comes to full boil. Remove from heat, and immediately add the chocolate and cocoa powder. Stir until the chocolate is melted. Add the bean mixture and stir until well-combined. Add the flour and stir until just combined. (Note: The batter will have a little texture to it if using whole chia seeds.)

4. Spread the batter into the prepared pan. Bake until springy to the touch, about 22 minutes. Remove from the oven. Cool completely in the pan on a rack. When cool, cut into 16 squares and serve. Or store in the refrigerator for up to 10 days or freezer for up to 3 months.

NUTRITION INFO

Choices/Exchanges: 1 starch, ½ carbohydrate, 1 fat

Per serving: 140 calories, 7 g total fat, 2 g saturated fat, 0 g trans fat, 0 mg cholesterol, 90 mg sodium, 148 mg potassium, 21 g total carbohydrate, 3 g dietary fiber, 13 g sugars, 12 g added sugars, 2 g protein, 39 mg phosphorus

Bean Bonus

You won't use an entire can of black beans for this recipe. What should you do with the rest? Save them with their liquid in a sealed glass jar or container in the refrigerator for up to 3 days. Use them in *Chilaquiles-Style Bowl* (page 69). Or drain them and toss with a little extra-virgin olive oil, red wine vinegar, and fresh herbs of choice for a quick-to-fix bean salad side dish anytime. Or, easier yet, sprinkle the desired amount of beans onto a leafy salad to punch up its protein.

NUTTY CANDY-BAR MINIS

Go ahead! Have a chewy, chocolatey candy bar. In fact, have two of them. I know, that sounds odd to tell someone with diabetes or prediabetes, but I'm referring to these mini bars. They actually have health benefits while still being totally candy-like with plenty of chocolatiness. The natural sweetness is mainly thanks to dates, since I suggest using no-sugar-added chocolate. And the rest of the body of the bars includes health-protective nuts and seeds. These minis are awesome as dessert, a snack, or whenever you just need a little oomph.

SERVES: 12 | SERVING SIZE: 2 mini bars
PREP TIME: 25 minutes (including freezing time) | COOK TIME: < 1 minute

- 6 ounces dried, pitted dates
- ⅓ cup shelled, salted, roasted pistachios or peanuts
- ⅓ cup shelled hemp seeds
- ⅓ cup creamy, natural, no-sugar-added peanut or almond butter
- 3 tablespoons unsweetened cocoa powder
- 1¼ teaspoons pure vanilla extract
- ⅛ teaspoon fine sea salt
- 3 ounces no-sugar-added (monk fruit- or stevia-sweetened) vegan baking chocolate (about 60% cacao), roughly chopped
- ¾ teaspoon unrefined coconut oil
- ⅛ teaspoon sea salt flakes

DIRECTIONS

1. In a food processor, blend the dates, pistachios or peanuts, hemp seeds, peanut or almond butter, cocoa powder, vanilla, and sea salt on low speed until well-combined and a dough forms but mixture still has some nutty texture.
2. Using clean hands, extra-firmly press the doughy mixture to form a 6-inch square on a silicone mat-lined small baking sheet or cutting board. Freeze for 10 minutes. Then transfer the square slab directly onto a cutting board, cut into 24 mini bars, and slightly separate each (so there's room to allow chocolate to drip down the sides of each mini bar).

3. In a small microwave-safe bowl, melt the chocolate with the coconut oil in the microwave, about 45 seconds to 1 minute (or use a double boiler).
4. Using a small spoon, drizzle then gently spread the top of each mini bar with the melted chocolate, letting it drip slightly down the sides of each. Then sprinkle with the sea salt flakes. Let stand at room temperature or the fridge until the chocolate coating is firm. Store in the fridge or freezer.

NUTRITION INFO

Choices/Exchanges: 1 fruit, ½ high fat protein, 1 fat

Per serving: 170 calories, 10 g total fat, 3 g saturated fat, 0 g trans fat, 0 mg cholesterol, 60 mg sodium, 268 mg potassium, 17 g total carbohydrate, 4 g dietary fiber, 9 g sugars, 0 g added sugars, 5 g protein, 117 mg phosphorus

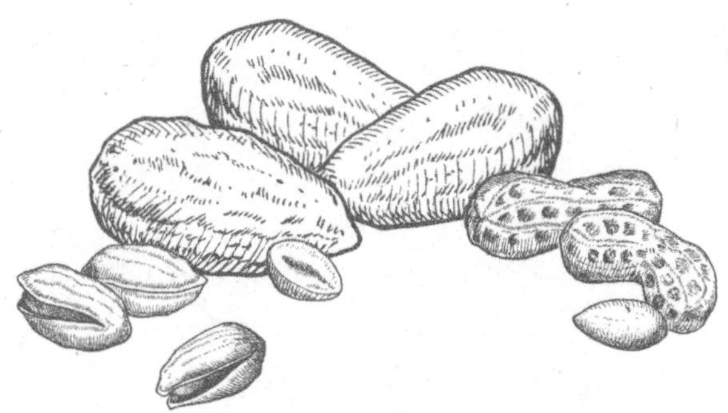

GRILLED FIGS WITH BALSAMIC REDUCTION

I adore fresh figs, especially in late summer. I often eat them all up before I actually gather up ingredients to use them in a recipe. But here's a recipe that I'm sure to save six fig beauties for. Be sure to do the same. Grilling the figs creates enticing caramelization. Finishing with a drizzling of a deep and distinctive balsamic vinegar reduction and a sprinkling of crunchy pistachios, this sweet and savory appetizer has amazing appeal.

SERVES: 4 | SERVING SIZE: 3 fig halves each
PREP TIME: 10 minutes | COOK TIME: 13 minutes

- ¼ cup aged (8 to 10 years) balsamic vinegar
- 6 fresh Black Mission or Striped Tiger figs, stemmed, halved lengthwise
- Organic oil cooking spray
- ⅛ teaspoon sea salt, or to taste
- 1 tablespoon lightly salted roasted pistachios, chopped
- 1 teaspoon chopped fresh rosemary leaves
- ¼ teaspoon freshly ground black pepper, or to taste

DIRECTIONS

1. Bring the vinegar to a boil in a small saucepan over high heat. Reduce heat to medium-low and simmer until the vinegar reduces by about half, about 7 minutes. Set aside to cool.
2. Prepare an outdoor or indoor grill or grill pan. Spritz the cut surface of each fig half with cooking spray (or extra-lightly brush with extra-virgin olive oil). Grill over direct, medium-high heat on the cut side until caramelized, about 3½ minutes.
3. Arrange the fig halves on a platter. Sprinkle with the salt and drizzle with desired amount of the balsamic reduction. Sprinkle with the pistachios, rosemary, and pepper. Serve at room temperature as a dessert—or a snack, appetizer, or side dish.

NUTRITION INFO
Choices/Exchanges: ½ fruit, ½ carbohydrate
Per serving: 80 calories, 1.5 g total fat, 0 g saturated fat, 0 g trans fat, 0 mg cholesterol, 85 mg sodium, 210 mg potassium, 18 g total carbohydrate, 2 g dietary fiber, 15 g sugars, 0 g added sugars, 1 g protein, 20 mg phosphorus

SUPERFRUITY SMOOTHIE

This fruity smoothie has "superfruity" benefits! Blueberries provide a punch of antioxidants, natural sweetness, and beautiful purplish color. Banana offers the nutritious creaminess. Lemon juice balances the taste along with providing its citrusy fragrance. And there's more. Unsweetened vanilla plant-based milk provides the dairy-like quality, and chia seeds add protein and texture intrigue. It's a slurpy snack or refreshing treat! (Hint: Buy several small bananas in advance, peel, break into four pieces each, and freeze; you'll be ready to whirl up this delightful smoothie anytime.)

SERVES: 2 | SERVING SIZE: about 1 cup
PREP TIME: 6 minutes (not including banana freezing time) | COOK TIME: 0 minutes

- 1 small banana, peeled, broken into four pieces, and frozen
- 1 cup frozen blueberries (do not thaw)
- ¾ cup unsweetened vanilla plant-based milk, chilled
- Juice of ½ small lemon (1 tablespoon)
- 2 teaspoons chia seeds

DIRECTIONS

1. Add all ingredients to a blender. Cover and purée until extra creamy, about 2 minutes on high speed.
2. Pour into glasses and serve.

NUTRITION INFO

Choices/Exchanges: 1½ fruit, ½ fat

Per serving: 120 calories, 2.5 g total fat, 0 g saturated fat, 0 g trans fat, 0 mg cholesterol, 70 mg sodium, 306 mg potassium, 24 g total carbohydrate, 5 g dietary fiber, 14 g sugars, 0 g added sugars, 2 g protein, 59 mg phosphorus

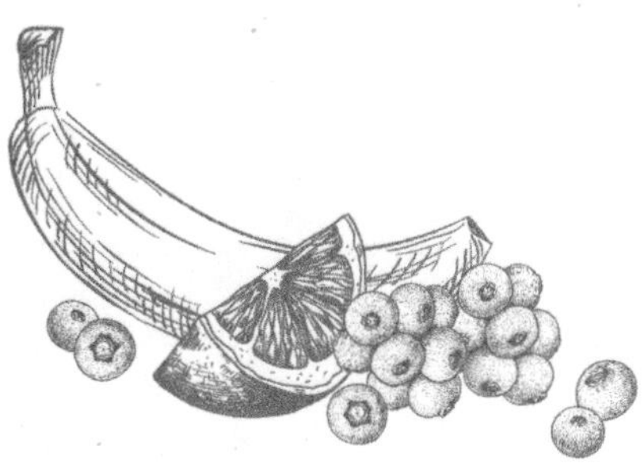

GREEN JUICE SMOOTHIE

Getting veggies into your eating plan—no matter how you do it—is a healthful goal. Drinking them is certainly one way to get them. By whirling the whole vegetables into a smoothie, you're still getting the full nutritional benefit of each, including all of the fiber. Here I've paired vegetables with fruit to give you bonus benefits and natural sweetness. The result is a vivid green, fragrant, and absolutely delightful beverage.

SERVES: 2 I SERVING SIZE: 1¼ cups
PREP TIME: 10 minutes I COOK TIME: 5 minutes (for brewing tea)

- 1¼ cups frozen mango cubes
- 1 cup chopped unpeeled English cucumber
- 1 cup packed fresh baby spinach or chopped chard
- ¾ cup unsweetened jasmine green tea (made with 1 tea bag) or filtered water, chilled
- 2 tablespoons packed fresh mint leaves
- Juice of ½ small lemon (1 tablespoon)
- 2 teaspoons fresh lime juice
- 1 teaspoon grated fresh gingerroot

DIRECTIONS

Purée all ingredients in a blender until smooth. Pour into 2 large beverage glasses and enjoy.

NUTRITION INFO

Choices/Exchanges: 1 fruit, 1 vegetable

Per serving: 80 calories, 0.5 g total fat, 0 g saturated fat, 0 g trans fat, 0 mg cholesterol, 15 mg sodium, 370 mg potassium, 19 g total carbohydrate, 2 g dietary fiber, 15 g sugars, 0 g added sugars, 2 g protein, 35 mg phosphorus

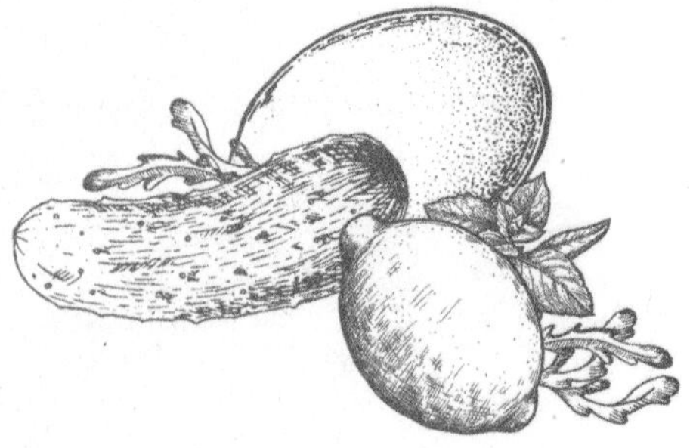

Glossary

Aquafaba	The liquid remaining from cooking chickpeas/garbanzo beans or other beans, often used as a replacement for egg whites or whole eggs in plant-based recipes
Aquafaba "mayo"	A vegan mayo made with sunflower oil, aquafaba, and seasonings
Arils	The small, round, juicy seeds inside pomegranates
Baba ghanoush	An Middle Eastern spread or dip based on eggplant and tahini
Chilaquiles	Traditional Mexican breakfast dish of fried corn tortillas simmered in salsa
Coconut aminos	Savory, soy-free sauce made from fermented coconut plant sap and seasonings that can be used like soy sauce
Crimini	Type of mushroom, also called baby bella mushroom
Farro	An ancient wheat grain with a chewy texture; it's a whole grain
FIFO	"First In, First Out," as in rotating pantry goods for freshness
Freekeh	A roasted, young, green durum wheat grain, also called farik; it's a whole grain
Gochujang	Fermented red chili paste used in Korean dishes
Harissa	Hot chili pepper and garlic paste from North Africa
Hoisin	A thick, Cantonese sauce used in stir-fries, to glaze meat, or for dipping
Kibbeh	A Middle Eastern food that typically includes ground meat, onions, bulgur wheat, and spices, such as cumin and mint
Korma	Indian curry dish made with meat, fish, or vegetables often braised in a yogurt mixture

Mizuna	Asian leafy green that can be used like arugula
Naan	A traditional flatbread originating from India
"Nooch"	Nickname for nutritional yeast flakes
Piperine	An alkaloid (naturally-occurring compound) that gives black pepper its "bite"
Pulses	Generally refers to dry beans, peas, chickpeas, and lentils
Quinoa	Nutrition-rich seeds from an Andean plant; they're considered "pseudograins"
Satay	Classically, Southeast Asian-seasoned, skewered, grilled meat served with sauce
Seitan	Plant protein-rich food made from wheat gluten, also called "wheat meat"
Soba noodles	Thin Japanese noodles traditionally made from buckwheat
Sumac	A deep red Middle Eastern spice with a tangy taste
Tahini	Sesame seed paste
Tamari	A wheat-free soy sauce that's a gluten-free alternative to typical soy sauce
Tatsoi	An Asian cruciferous vegetable with leafy greens, similar to bok choy
Teff	A powerhouse whole-grain seed from an ancient African grass
Tempeh	Fermented soybean "cake"—it's savory, not sweet
Tofunnaise	A condiment similar to mayonnaise that's based on tofu
Tree nuts	Includes almonds, Brazil nuts, cashews, hazelnuts, macadamia nuts, pecans, pine nuts, pistachios, and walnuts
Tzatziki	Yogurt and cucumber dip or sauce
Umami	One of our senses of taste that's savory or meaty
"Wheat meat"	See seitan

Index

C

T

About the Author

Jackie Newgent, RDN, CDN, sure has come a long way since her earliest childhood creation of bologna-potato chip canapés. She's passionate about plant-based cuisine and the environment—and a lifelong fan of flavorful food. Her mantra is: Go for great taste; aim for plant-based; try not to waste.

Jackie is a plant-forward registered dietitian nutritionist, classically trained chef, award-winning cookbook author, professional recipe developer, media personality, spokesperson, and food writer. She's the author of six cookbooks, including *The All-Natural Diabetes Cookbook, 1,000 Low-Calorie Recipes, The Clean & Simple Diabetes Cookbook, The With or Without Meat Cookbook,* and *Big Green Cookbook.*

Jackie is a Forbes Health advisory board member and a private plant-based cooking coach. She advises start-up food companies on product development. Jackie has made guest appearances on dozens of television news shows, including *Good Morning America.* Formerly, she was a healthy cooking instructor at the Institute of Culinary Education for about twenty years and a national media spokesperson for the Academy of Nutrition and Dietetics.

Jackie is based in Brooklyn, New York, where she is also co-founder of Peterra Kitchen, a plant-forward pet treat company, which was inspired by her cat, Baby Duke. In her free time, Jackie loves to get out into nature, including hiking and kayaking.

Follow her on social media: @jackienewgent. For Jackie's plant-based recipe blog and more information about her, visit jackienewgent.com.